TRAUMA HEALING JOURNAL

FOR WOMEN

GENTLE

Strength

A 12-WEEK RECOVERY WORKBOOK FOR INNER STABILITY, HEALING AND POSITIVE TRANSFORMATION

BY CHLOÉ GRAYSON

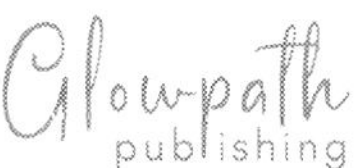

Gentle Strength: Trauma Healing Journal For Women

ISBN: 978-3-911105-01-9

Herausgeber: Renate Klysch - Berlin

FIRST EDITION: 2023

Published by Glowpath Publishing

Introduction

Welcome to your personal trauma healing journal.

This is a safe and supportive space personally designed for women like you who are on a journey towards healing and growth. It will help you as you compassionately and tenderly delve into the deepest parts of your feelings, thoughts, and experiences.

Us women often encounter a variety of unique challenges throughout our lives, such as traumatic experiences that can make us question the way we see ourselves, our relationships, and our values. However, none of these effects should ever keep you from being the person you were meant to be. You are the creator of your own story, and any hardship can be turned into a source of tremendous strength and growth.

This journal is a judgement-free zone. It's never necessary to compare your progress to that of other people, and there are no right or wrong answers. Your unique experiences and feelings are valid and important, and examining them through writing can be an incredibly powerful process.

Please be kind to yourself as you start upon this journey. As women, it is all too easy for us to take things to heart, beat ourselves up for mistakes (even the ones we didn't make) and hold on to negative emotions and thoughts. Helping you finally let go of all of that is the goal of this journal. Try to be as compassionate and gentle with yourself as possible. You deserve patience and kindness as you go through this process. Treat yourself the way you would treat a close friend.

This journal is divided into 12 stages, one for each week. They will gently guide you toward a better understanding of what transpired and how you can move on from it. Thoughtfully designed to address the many crucial elements of your healing process, the prompts you'll come across include delving into the trauma itself, processing negative feelings, recognizing triggers, establishing personal boundaries, and cultivating self-compassion.

Every journal entry you make will serve as a stepping stone towards your beautiful transformation. And even though the order of these prompts has been carefully curated to create the most beneficial experience for you, remember that this journal is all yours. You may not feel ready to answer certain questions right away and that's completely okay. Or you may decide that you would rather open the book at a random page and make that your entry for the day. Everything is allowed. You can't do anything wrong.

Once you delve into the healing process, remember that you are never alone. Countless women have been through similar struggles and triumphed over their traumas, just as you will. Celebrate your progress, no matter how small it seems. Healing is not just measured by massive breakthroughs (which you will undoubtedly encounter) but by your willingness to show up for yourself. One journal entry at a time.

You are not defined by your trauma but by your resilience and strength in the face of it. Embrace the transformative power of writing.

Be the creator of your own story.

WEEK 1

Setting Intentions & Establishing Safety

In this first week you will embark on your personal healing journey with purpose and care. You will set empowering intentions and explore your motivations for healing and growth. You can let your guard down and express yourself without fear of repercussions by creating a nurturing and safe environment. Your trauma healing journal will become a place of refuge where you can recognize your resilience and clear the path for a successful future.

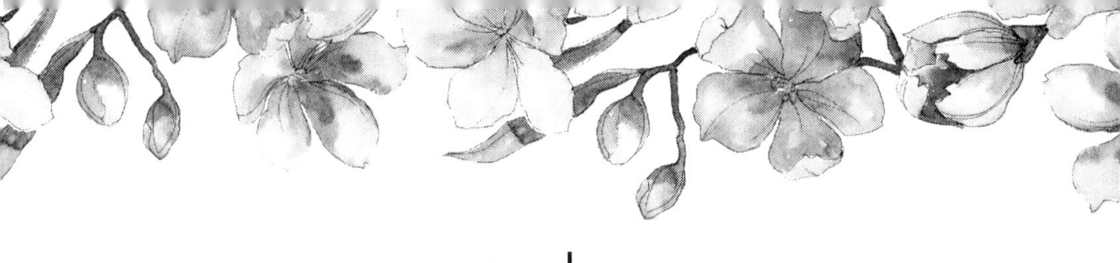

WEEK 1 | DAY 1

WHAT ARE YOUR INTENTIONS FOR THIS HEALING JOURNEY? WHAT ARE YOUR HOPES AND EXPECTATIONS?

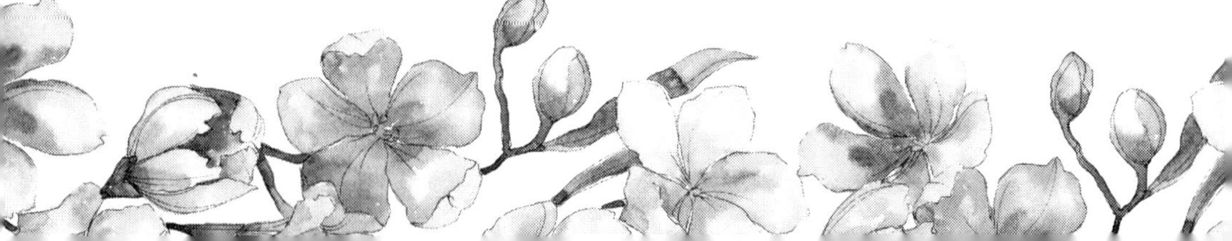

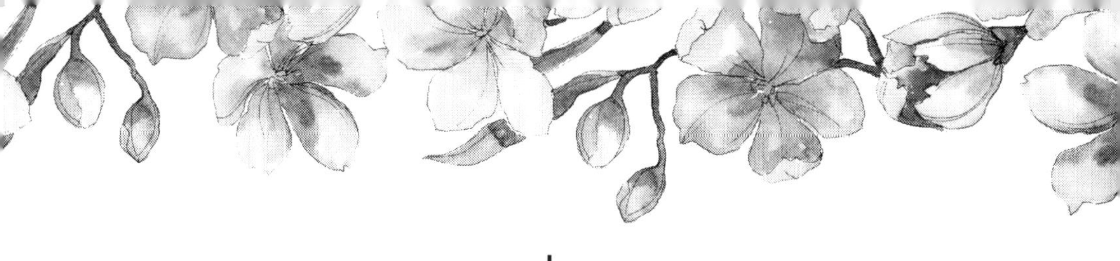

WEEK 1 | DAY 2

WHAT DOES YOU SAFE SPACE LOOK LIKE?

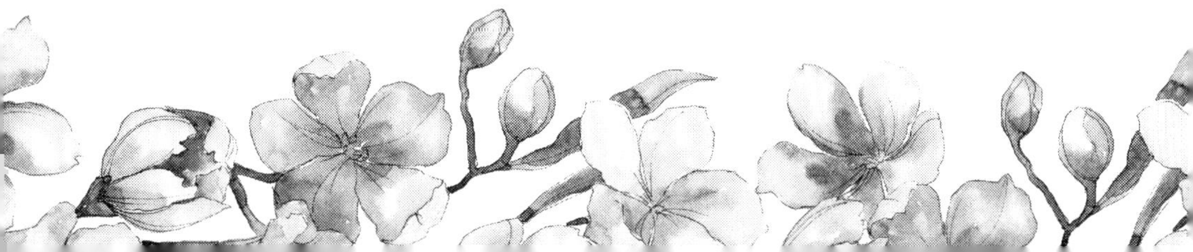

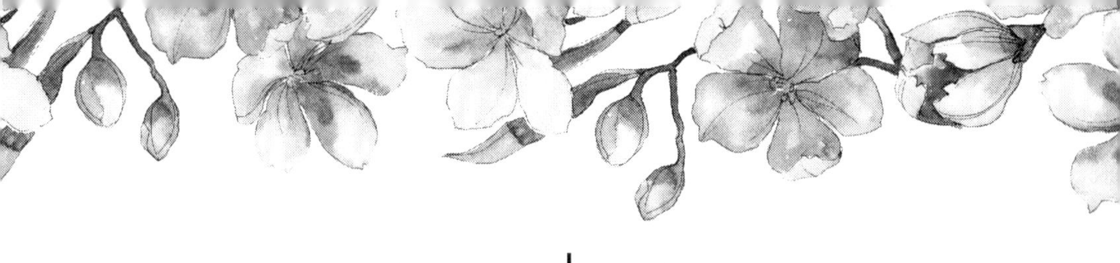

WEEK 1 | DAY 3

DO YOU HAVE ANY SPECIFIC FEARS OR HESITATIONS ABOUT EXPLORING YOUR TRAUMA THROUGH WRITING?

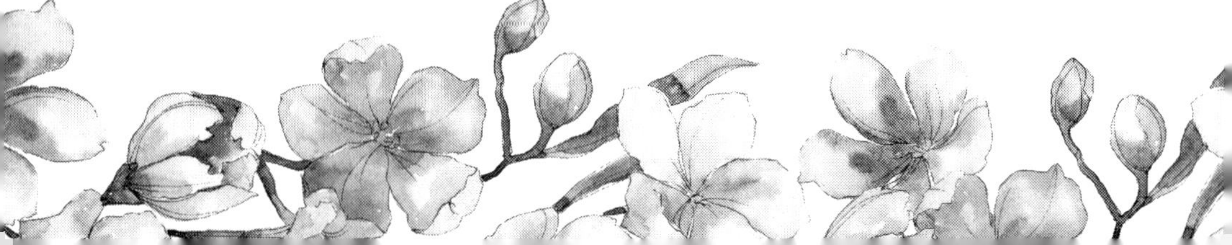

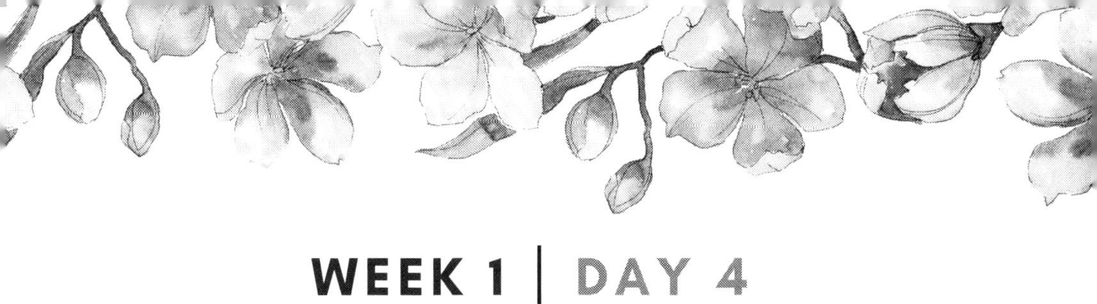

WEEK 1 | DAY 4

WHAT SELF-CARE PRACTICES CAN YOU INCORPORATE BEFORE AND AFTER YOUR JOURNALING SESSION TO ENSURE THAT YOU FEEL SAFE AND SECURE DURING THIS PROCESS?

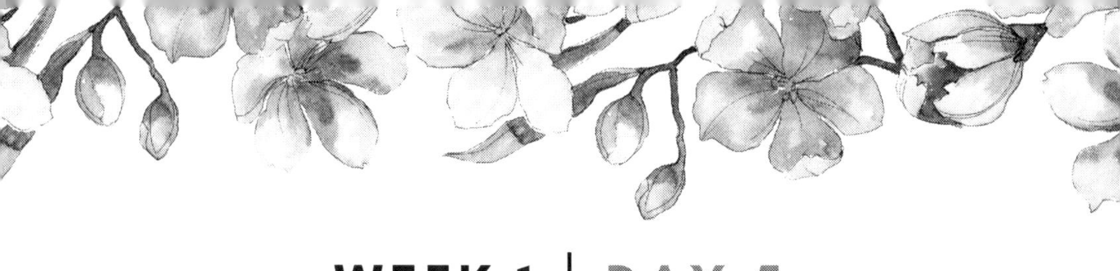

WEEK 1 | DAY 5

WRITE A LETTER OF COMPASSION TO YOUR PAST SELF:

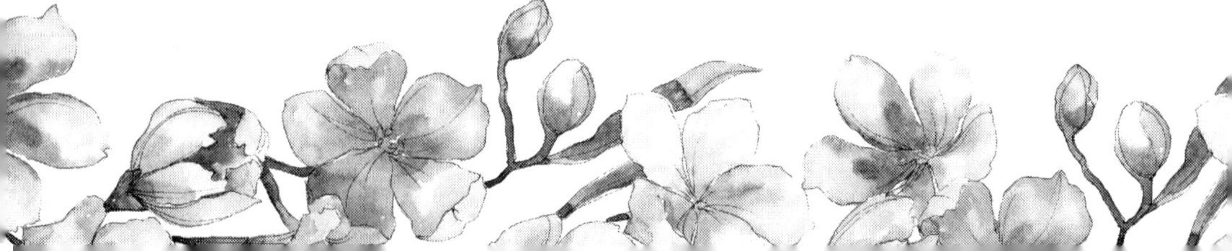

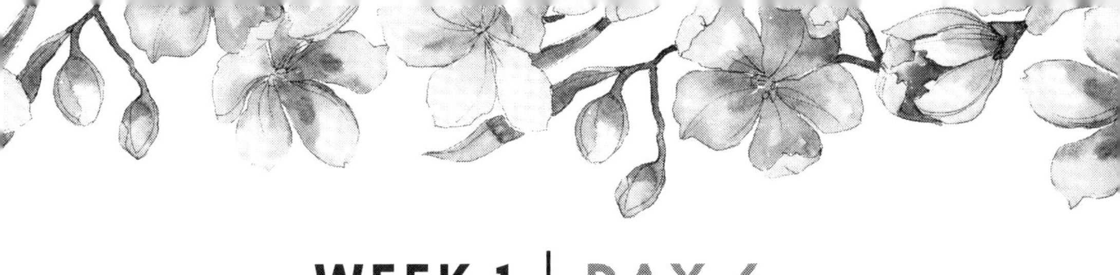

WEEK 1 | DAY 6

HOW CAN YOU BE AS KIND AND GENTLE AS POSSIBLE WITH YOURSELF AS YOU GO THROUGH THIS PROCESS?

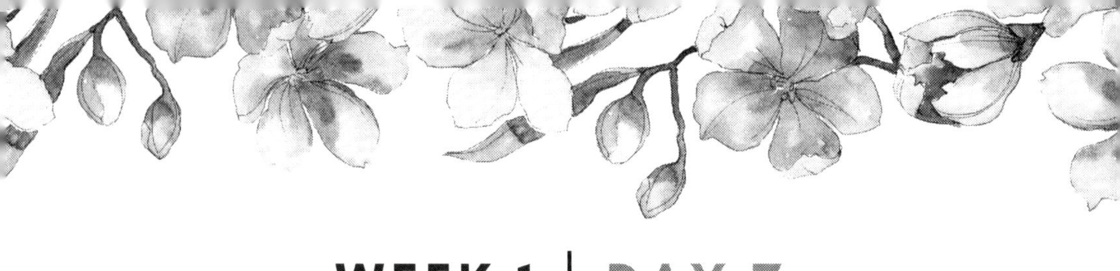

WEEK 1 | DAY 7

ACKNOWLEDGE THE COURAGE IT TAKES TO EMBARK ON THIS KIND OF HEALING JOURNEY. WRITE ABOUT THE STRENGTH YOU ALREADY POSSESS WITHIN YOU:

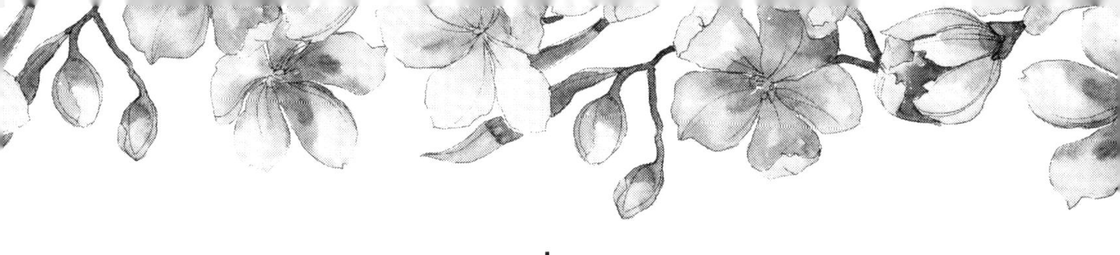

WEEK 1 | RECAP

HOW HAS THIS WEEK BEEN FOR YOU?

IN WHAT WAYS HAVE YOU GROWN?

WHAT COULD YOU DO BETTER NEXT WEEK?

WEEK 2

Revisiting Early Life

This week you will explore some of your early life experiences. You will reflect on your upbringing and childhood, and examine how past events have shaped your beliefs and emotions. By understanding your past you will gain greater clarity in your healing process. You will be able to honor your inner child and create the groundwork for significant personal development and transformation with each journal entry.

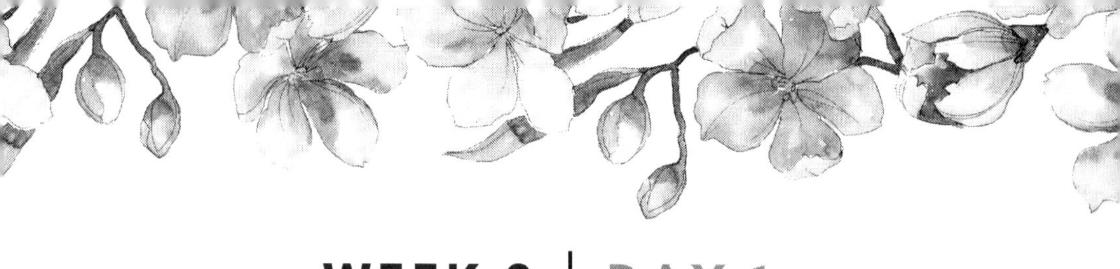

WEEK 2 | DAY 1

DESCRIBE YOUR EARLIEST MEMORIES AS A CHILD. HOW DOES THINKING BACK ON THEM MAKE YOU FEEL?

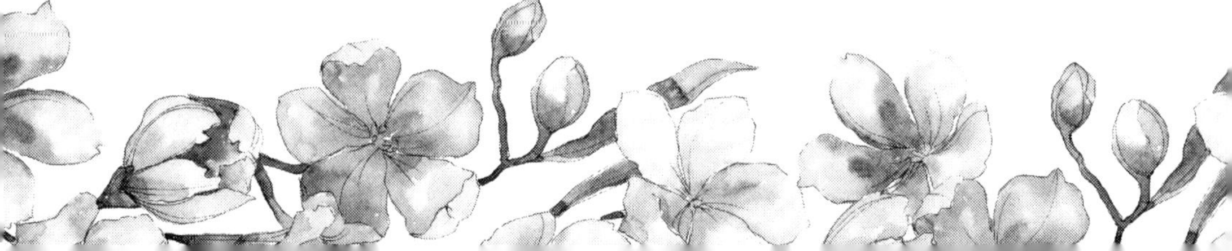

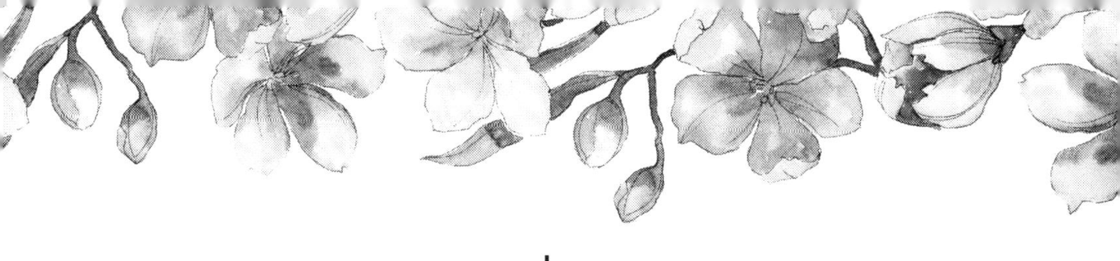

WEEK 2 | DAY 2

WHAT WERE YOUR FAMILY DYNAMICS LIKE? HOW DID YOUR PARENTS INTERACT WITH YOU? HOW DID THEY INTERACT WITH EACH OTHER?

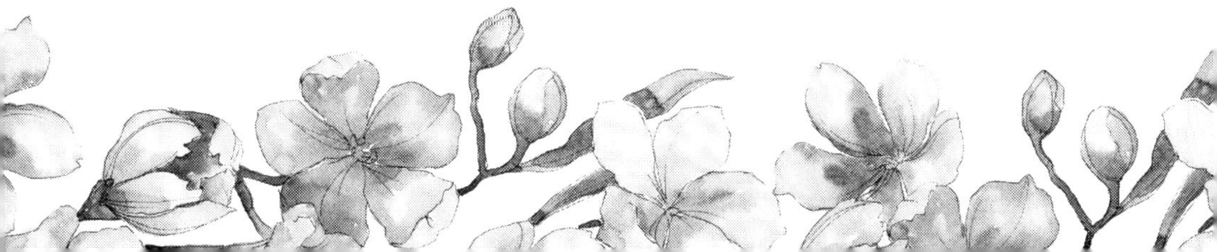

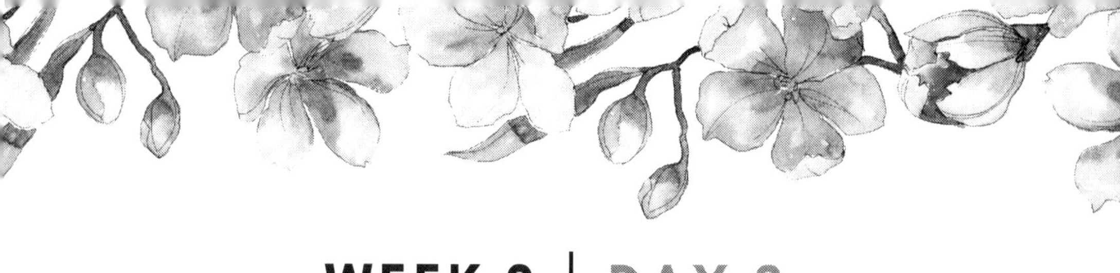

WEEK 2 | DAY 3

HOW DID YOU PROCESS EMOTIONS AS A CHILD?

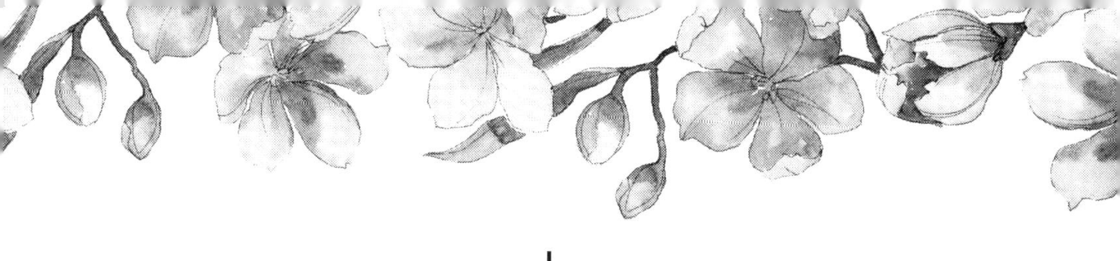

WEEK 2 | DAY 4

WRITE ABOUT A CHILDHOOD EVENT THAT HAD A SIGNIFICANT IMPACT ON YOU:

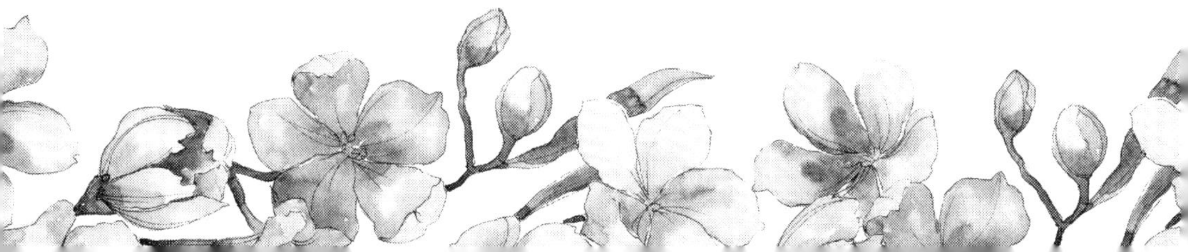

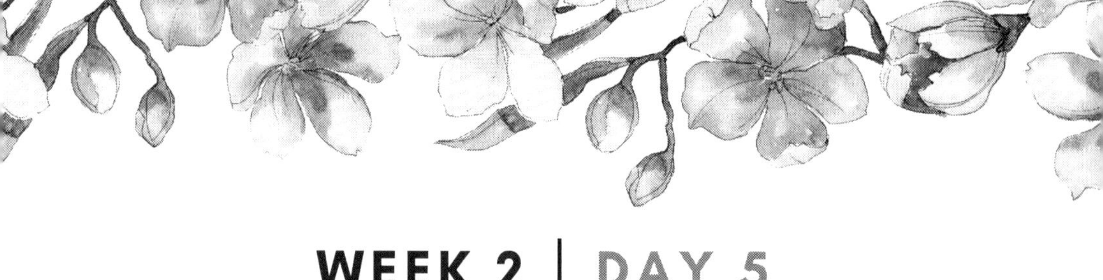

WEEK 2 | DAY 5

WHAT KINDS OF MESSAGES DID YOU RECEIVE ABOUT BEING VULNERABLE AND SHOWING EMOTION GROWING UP? HOW HAVE THESE MESSAGES SHAPED YOU AS AN ADULT?

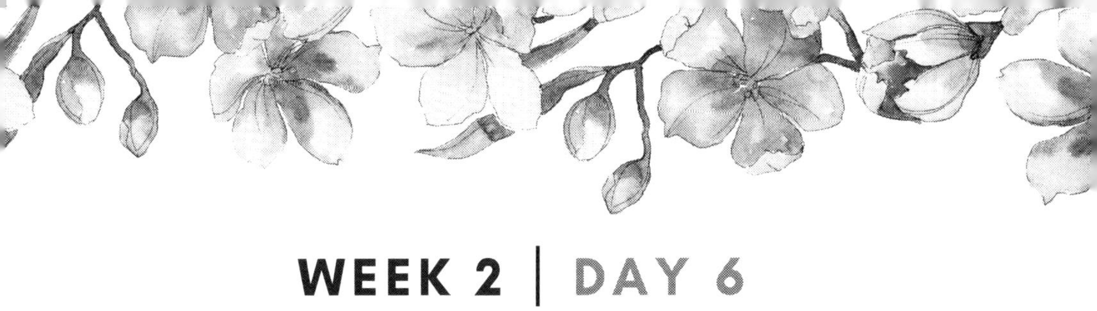

WEEK 2 | DAY 6

THINK BACK ON ANY EARLY EXPERIENCES WITH TRAUMA OR ADVERSITY. DID THESE THINGS LEAVE ANY LASTING IMPRESSIONS? DID SIMILAR THEMES SHOW UP AGAIN LATER?

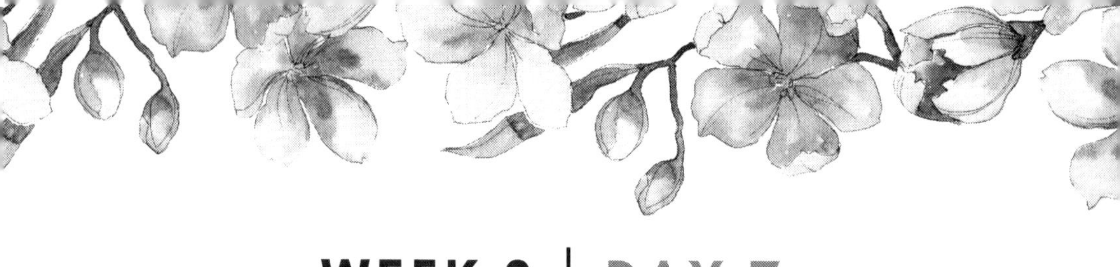

WEEK 2 | DAY 7

WHAT WERE THE THINGS THAT MADE YOU FEEL SAFE AND TAKEN CARE OF AS A CHILD?

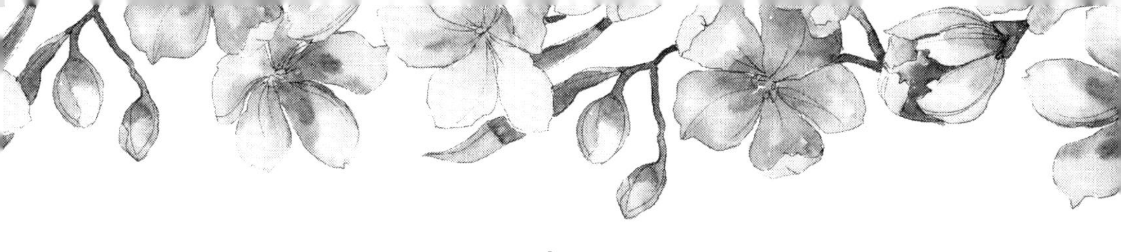

WEEK 2 | RECAP

HOW HAS THIS WEEK BEEN FOR YOU?

IN WHAT WAYS HAVE YOU GROWN?

WHAT COULD YOU DO BETTER NEXT WEEK?

WEEK 3

Exploring Traumatic Experiences

In this pivotal stage of your trauma healing journey you will bravely confront and explore your past traumatic experiences. Through self-compassion and empathy, you will start to peel back the layers of trauma that have affected your life. Even though it can seem like a difficult process at times, you will gain crucial understanding and clarity which are necessary for healing and transformation, by bringing these painful memories to light. Reclaim your narrative and seize this chance to accept your inner strength.

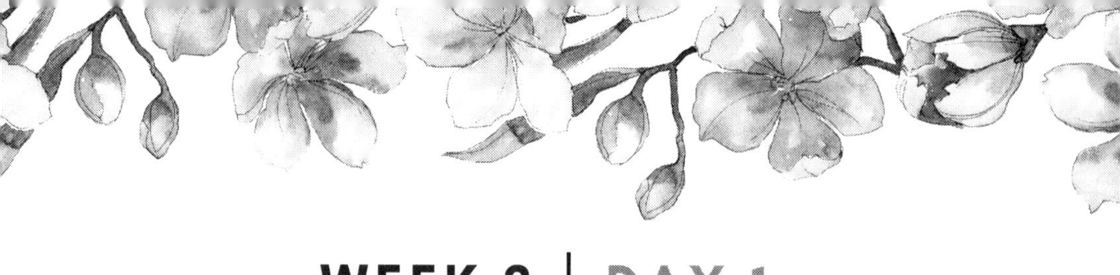

WEEK 3 | DAY 1

DESCRIBE THE TRAUMATIC EXPERIENCE YOU WOULD LIKE TO WORK THROUGH. BE AS SPECIFIC AS YOU WOULD LIKE TO BE, OR AS VAGUE AS YOU NEED TO BE:

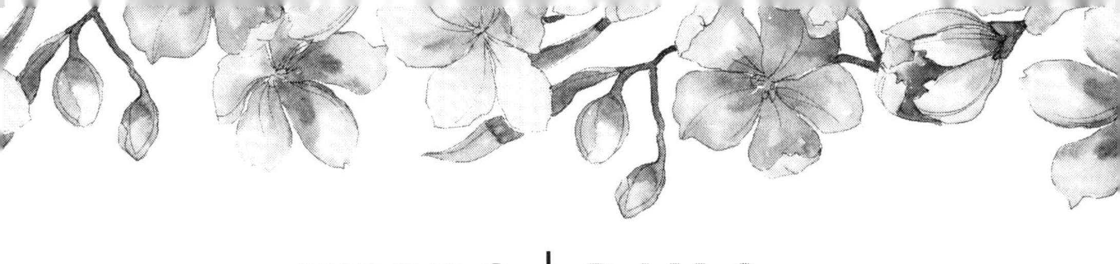

WEEK 3 | DAY 2

WHAT WERE YOUR DOMINANT FEELINGS AND EMOTIONS AS YOU WERE EXPERIENCING THIS?

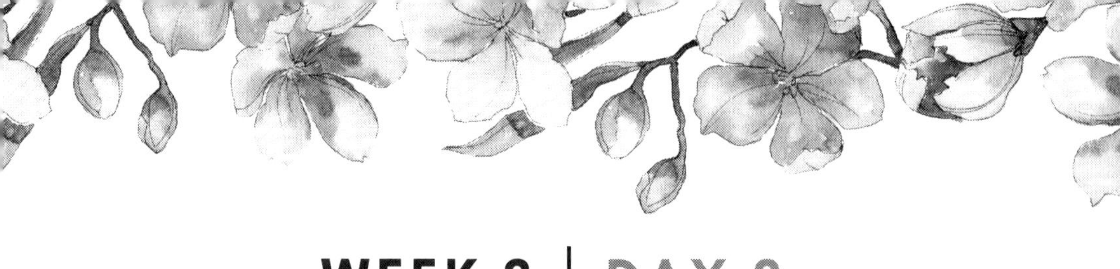

WEEK 3 | DAY 3

DID YOU REALIZE YOU WERE GOING THROUGH TRAUMA AS IT WAS HAPPENING? IF NOT, WHEN DID YOU?

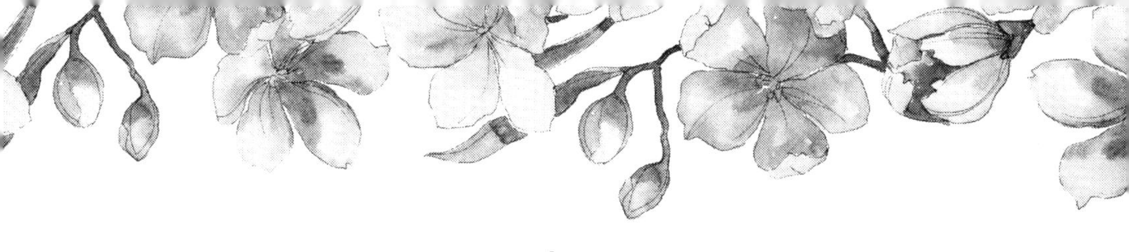

WEEK 3 | DAY 4

ARE THERE ANY ASPECTS OF YOUR EXPERIENCE THAT YOU HAVE BEEN AVOIDING OR SUPPRESSING?

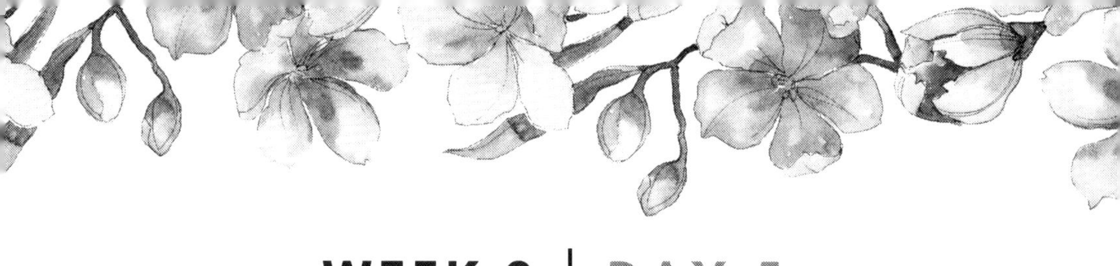

WEEK 3 | DAY 5

WHAT CHANGES HAVE YOU NOTICED IN YOURSELF EVER SINCE GOING THROUGH YOUR TRAUMA?

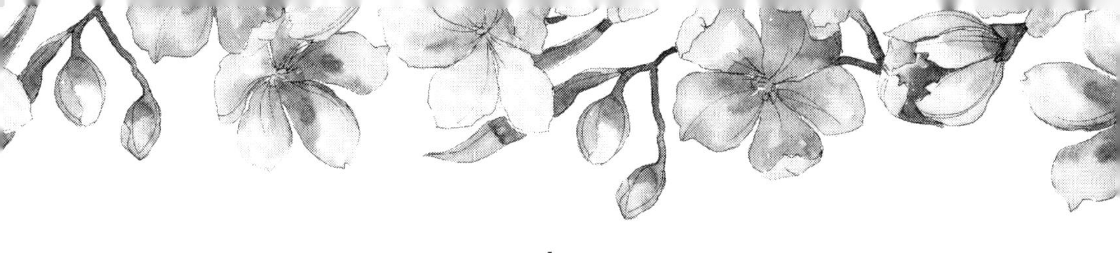

WEEK 3 | DAY 6

HAS YOUR PERSPECTIVE ON WHAT HAPPENED TO YOU CHANGED OVER TIME?

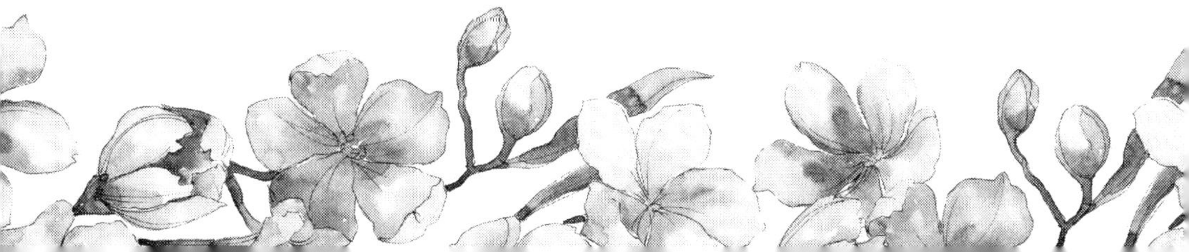

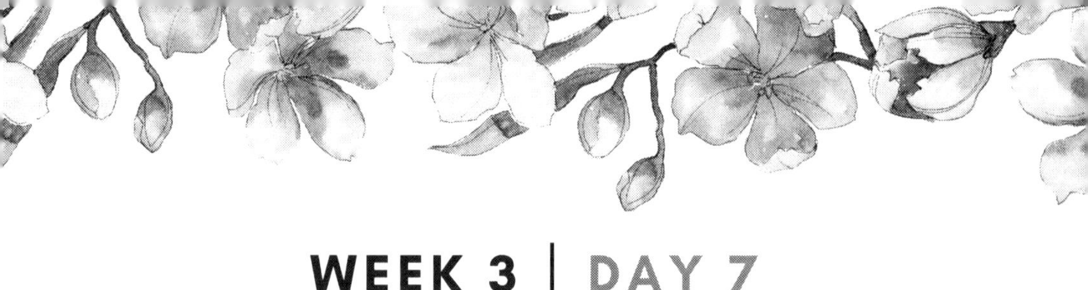

WEEK 3 | DAY 7

DO YOU SOMETIMES THINK ABOUT WHAT YOUR LIFE WOULD BE LIKE IF YOU HADN'T EXPERIENCED THIS TRAUMA? HOW DO THOSE THOUGHTS MAKE YOU FEEL?

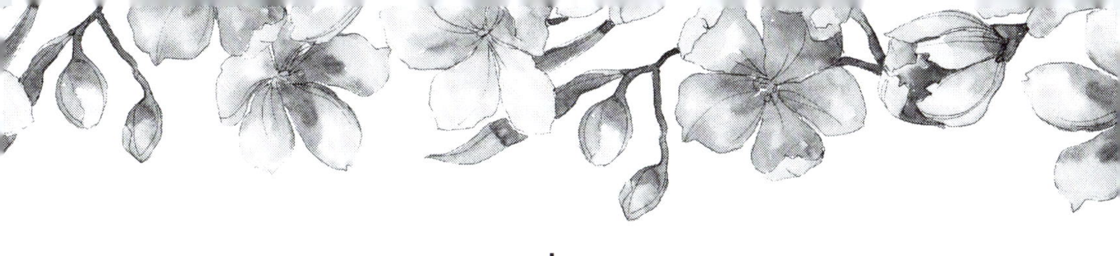

WEEK 3 | RECAP

HOW HAS THIS WEEK BEEN FOR YOU?

IN WHAT WAYS HAVE YOU GROWN?

WHAT COULD YOU DO BETTER NEXT WEEK?

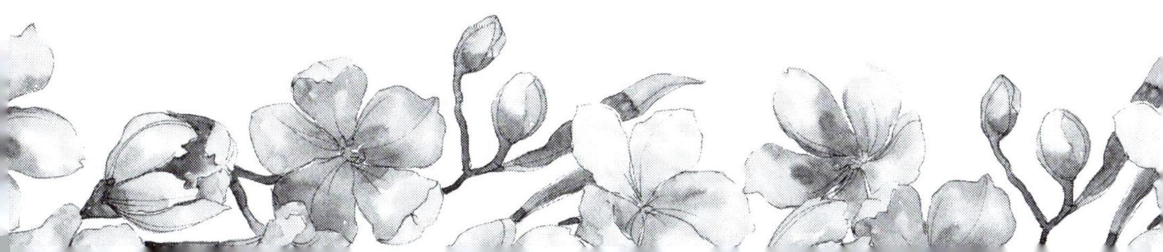

WEEK 4

Acknowledging Emotions

This week you will dive deep into the realm of emotions. You will be exploring the full spectrum of your feelings with gentle self-awareness and acceptance. Through heartfelt journaling, you will courageously acknowledge the emotions that have been long suppressed or overlooked, and allow yourself to feel and validate your emotional experiences without judgment.

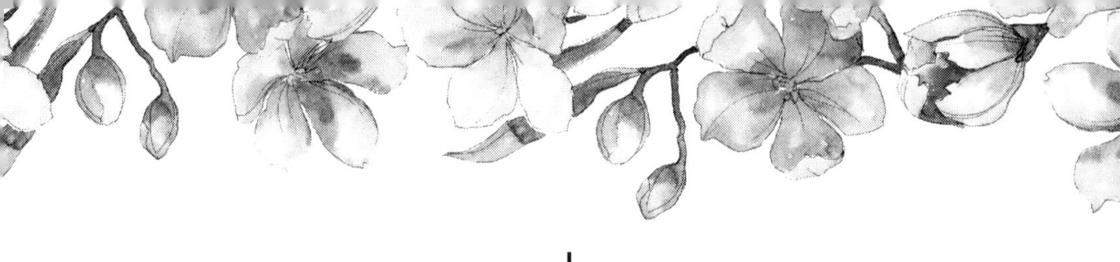

WEEK 4 | DAY 1

WHAT NEGATIVE EMOTIONS FROM THE PAST HAVE YOU BEEN HOLDING ON TO?

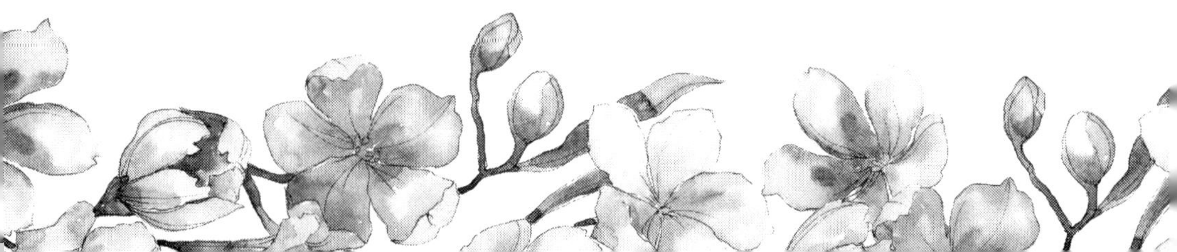

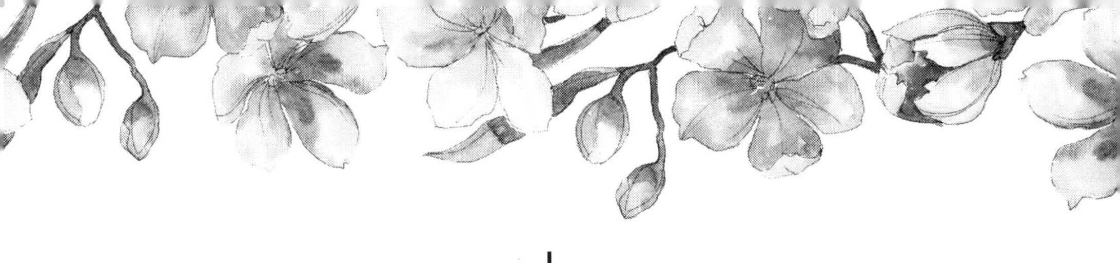

WEEK 4 | DAY 2

DO YOU SOMETIMES DOWNPLAY WHAT YOU'VE EXPERIENCED?

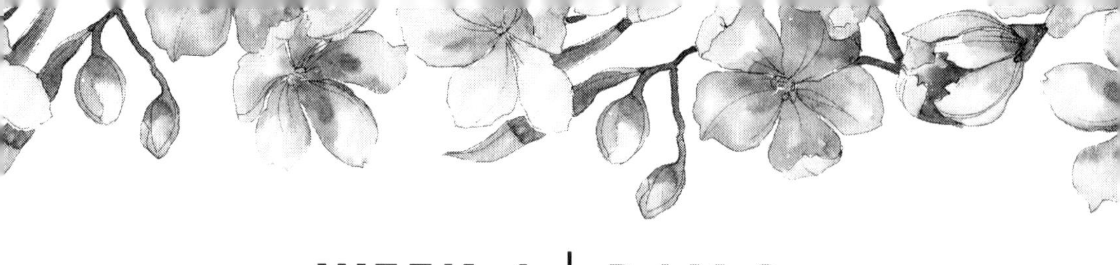

WEEK 4 | DAY 3

ARE YOU HOLDING ON TO ANY GUILT OR SHAME RELATED TO YOUR TRAUMA?

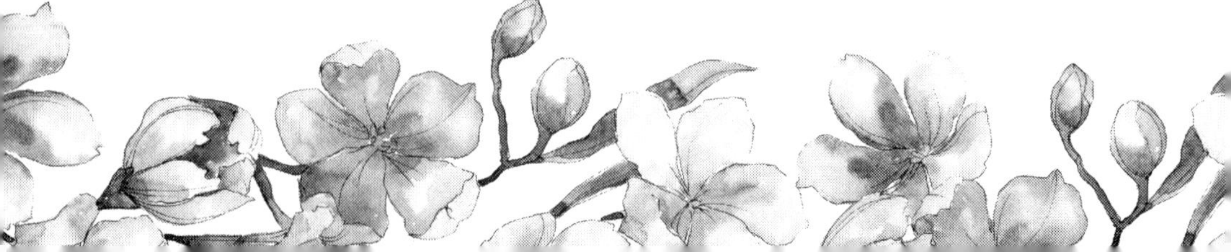

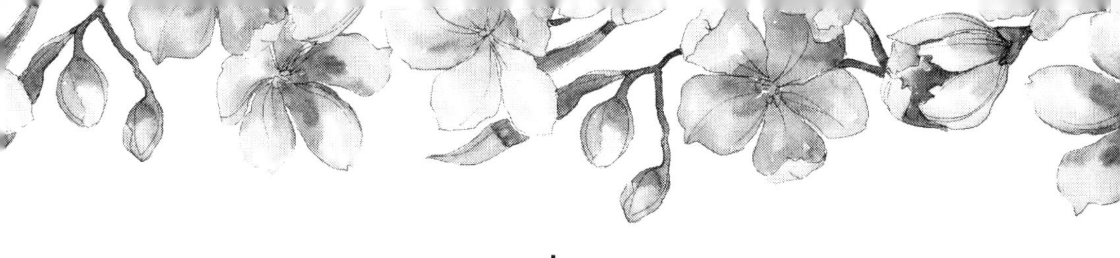

WEEK 4 | DAY 4

ARE THERE ANY RECURRING EMOTIONS YOU HAVE BEEN EXPERIENCING LATELY?

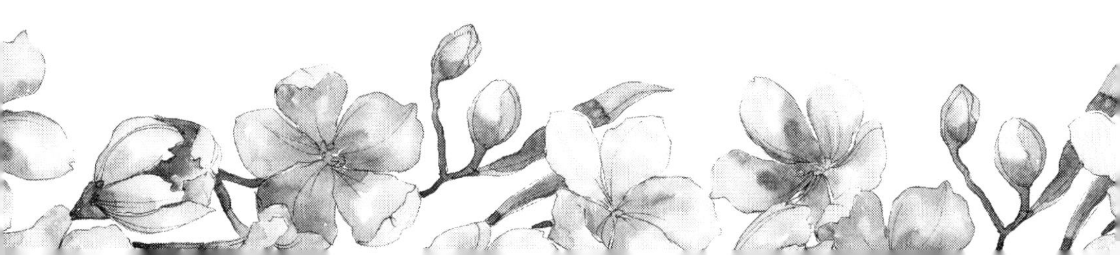

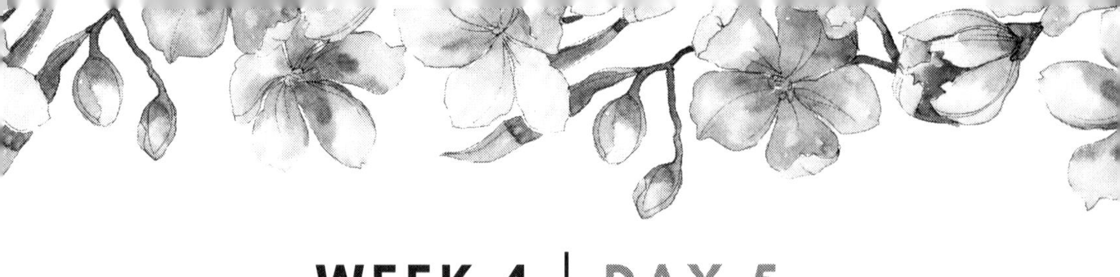

WEEK 4 | DAY 5

CAN YOU DESCRIBE A MOMENT OF EMOTIONAL RELEASE OR CATHARSIS THAT YOU'VE EXPERIENCED?

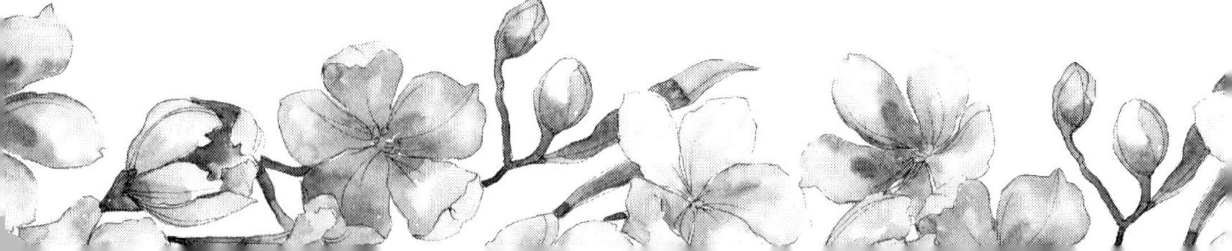

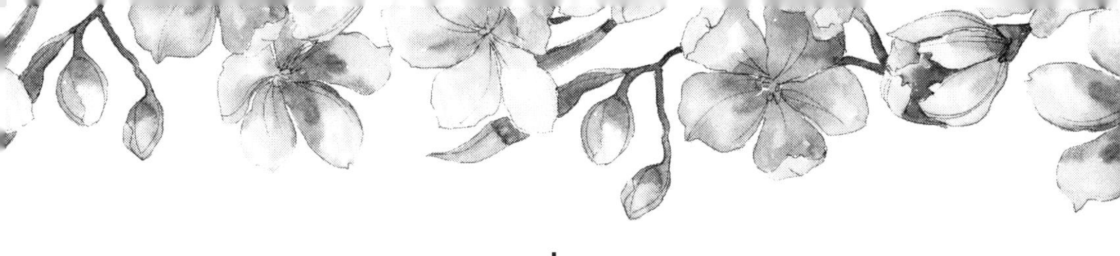

WEEK 4 | DAY 6

DO YOU FEEL ANY UNRESOLVED GRIEF OR LOSS RELATED TO YOUR TRAUMA?

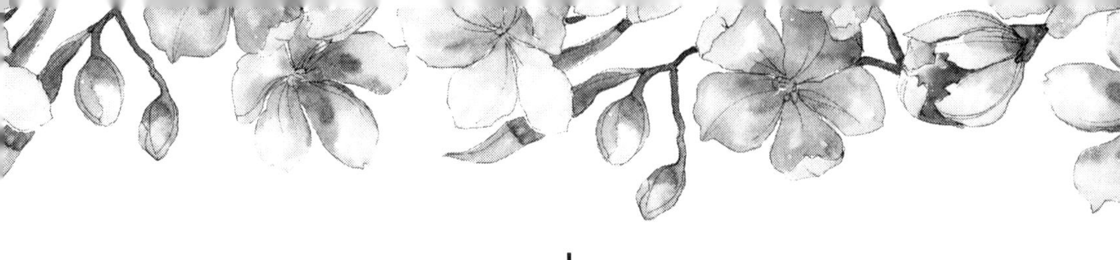

WEEK 4 | DAY 7

WHO OR WHAT MAKES YOU FEEL FULLY ACCEPTED AND UNDERSTOOD?

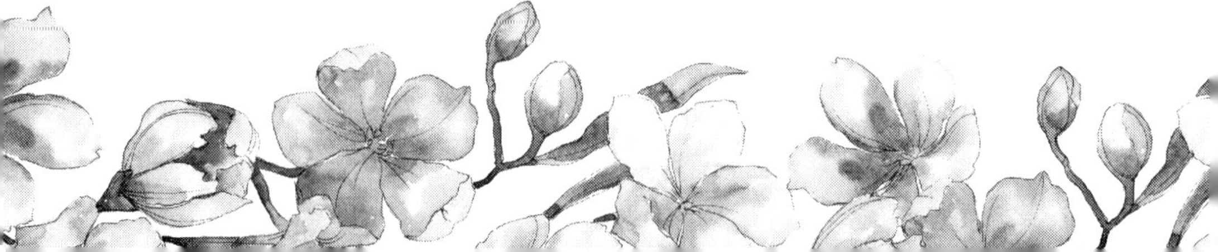

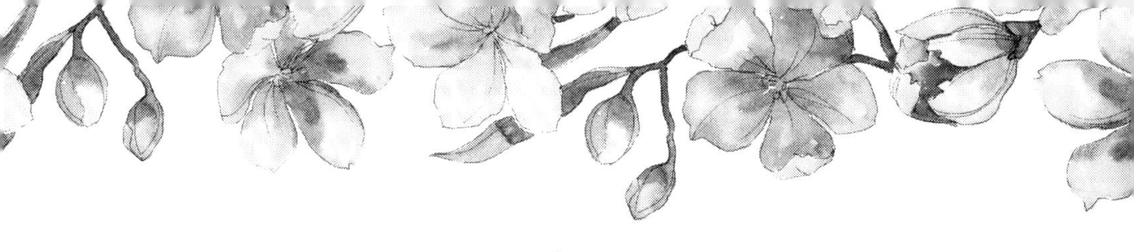

WEEK 4 | RECAP

HOW HAS THIS WEEK BEEN FOR YOU?

IN WHAT WAYS HAVE YOU GROWN?

WHAT COULD YOU DO BETTER NEXT WEEK?

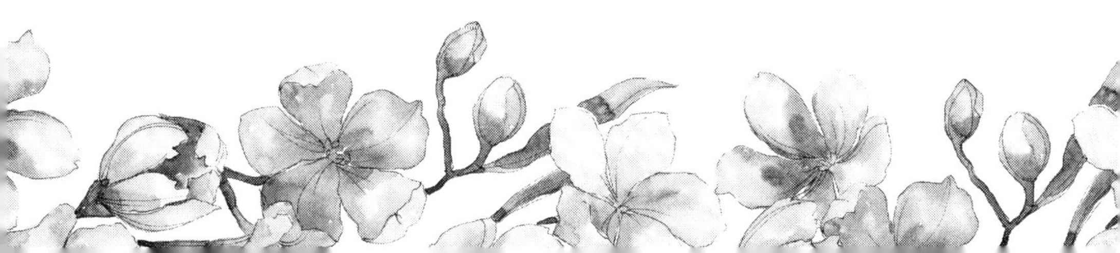

WEEK 5

Identifying Triggers & Patterns

In this stage of your healing journey you will identify the triggers and patterns that have shaped your responses to certain situations and relationships. The fundamental causes of your emotional responses and recurrent behaviors will become clear to you. You will be able to free yourself from their influence and take back control of your responses by being aware of these patterns and triggers.

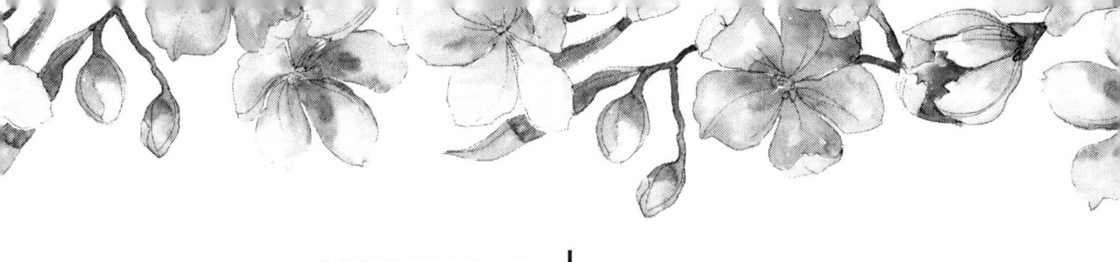

WEEK 5 | DAY 1

WHAT ARE THE MOST COMMON TRIGGERS FOR YOU? WHAT EMOTIONAL RESPONSES DO THEY EVOKE IN YOU?

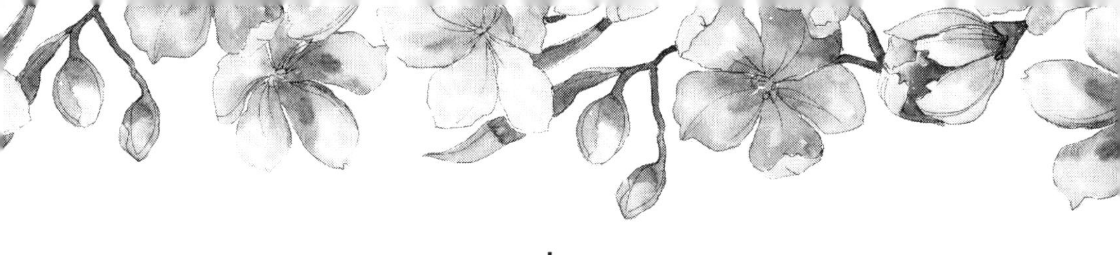

WEEK 5 | DAY 2

WHAT IS A NEGATIVE THOUGHT PATTERN THAT YOU WOULD LIKE TO CHANGE?

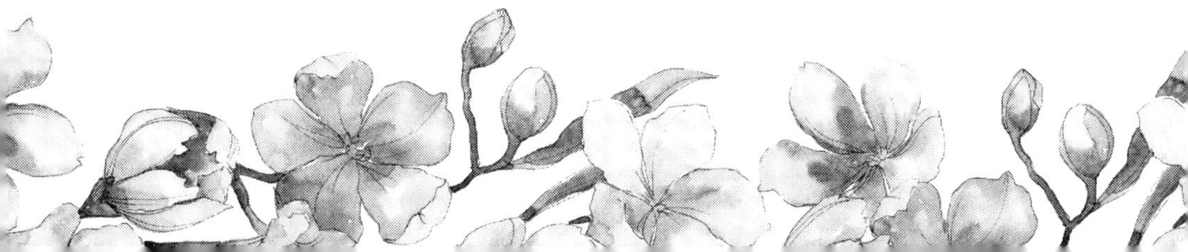

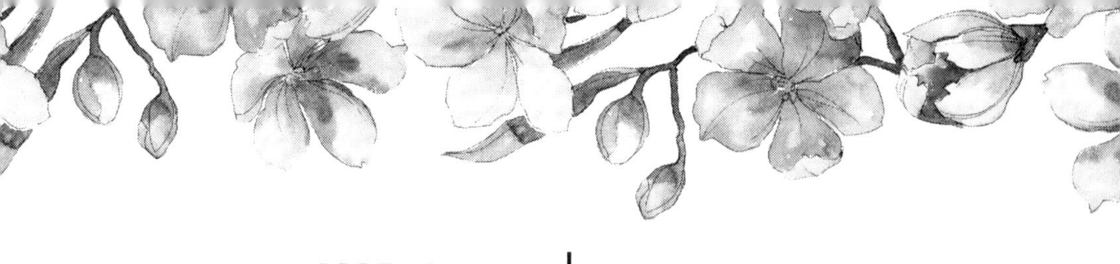

WEEK 5 | DAY 3

WHAT ARE THE USUAL PHYSICAL SENSATIONS YOU EXPERIENCE WHEN YOU ARE ANXIOUS OR STRESSED?

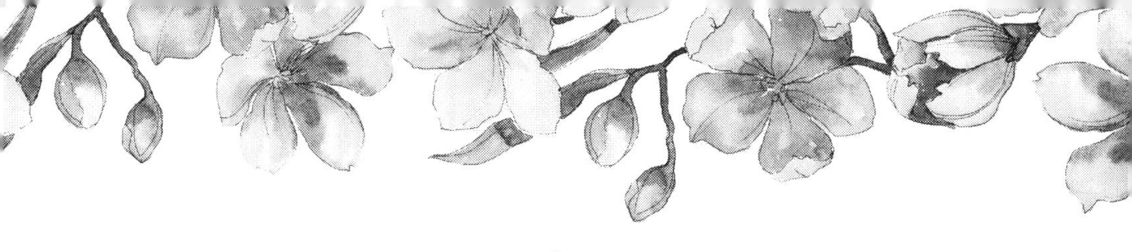

WEEK 5 | DAY 4

DID YOU DEVELOP ANY ADDICTIVE HABITS SINCE EXPERIENCING TRAUMA?

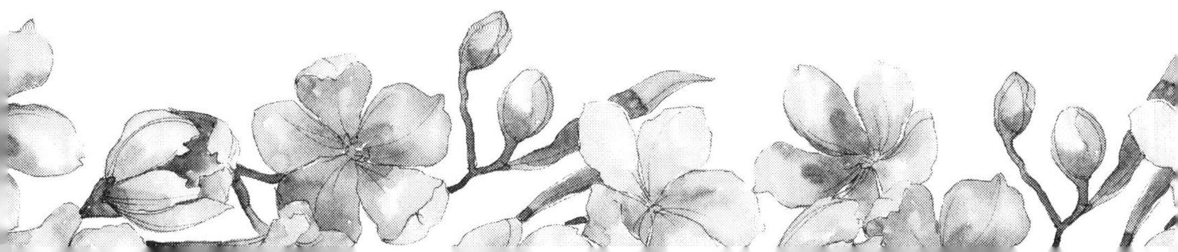

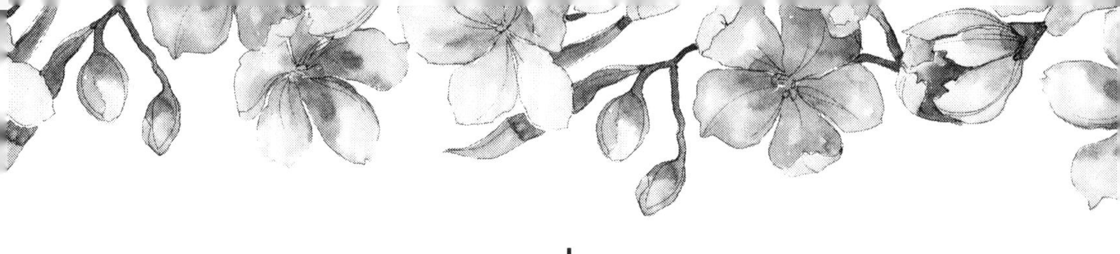

WEEK 5 | DAY 5

WHAT ARE SOME FEARS AND ANXIETIES YOU FEEL RELATED TO YOUR EXPERIENCE?

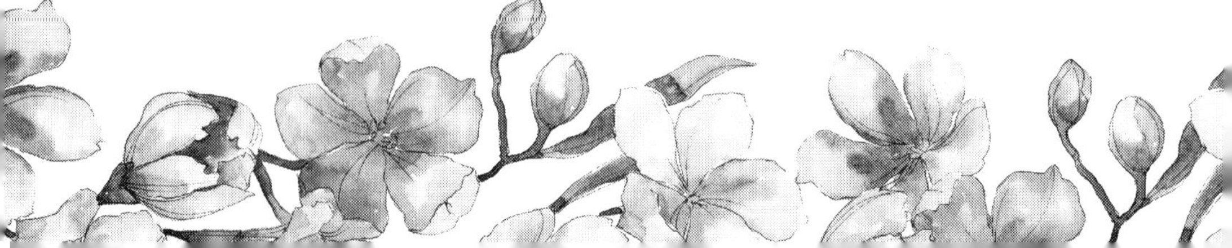

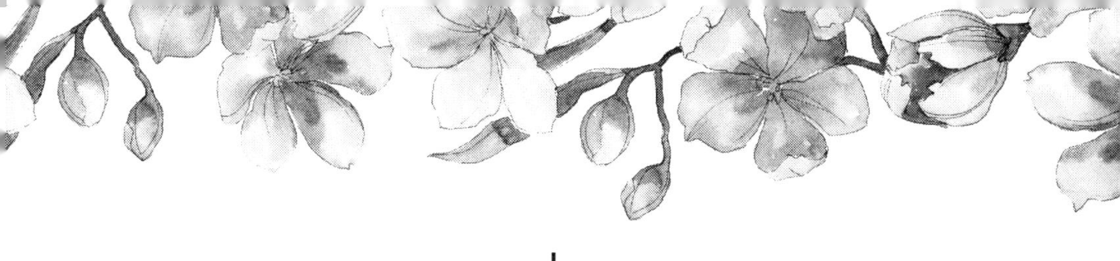

WEEK 5 | DAY 6

HAVE YOU EXPERIENCED ANY RECURRING DREAMS OR NIGHTMARES RELATED TO YOUR TRAUMA?

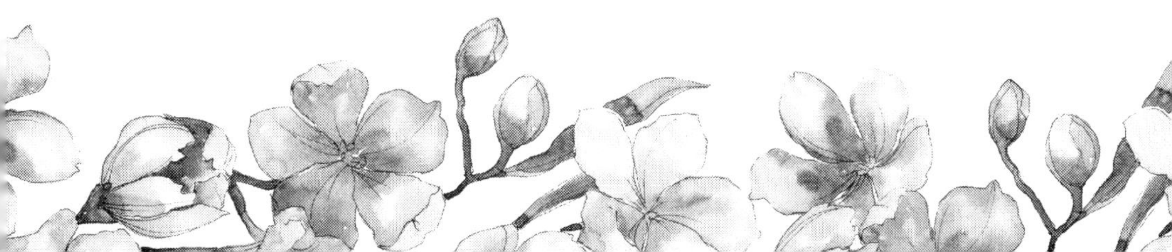

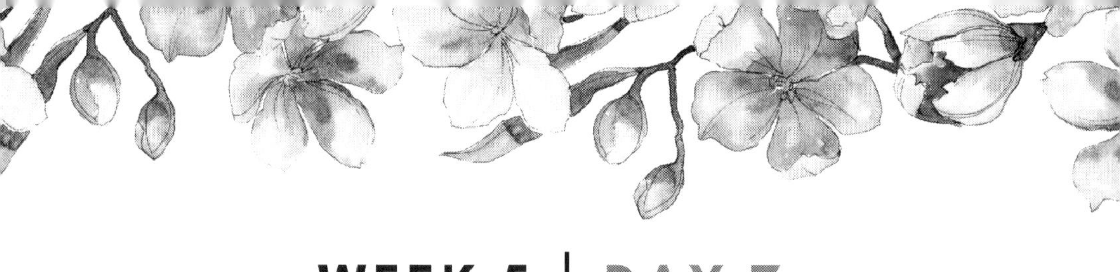

WEEK 5 | DAY 7

WRITE ABOUT A SITUATION IN WHICH YOU FELT TRIGGERED OR OVERWHELMED DUE TO YOUR TRAUMA:

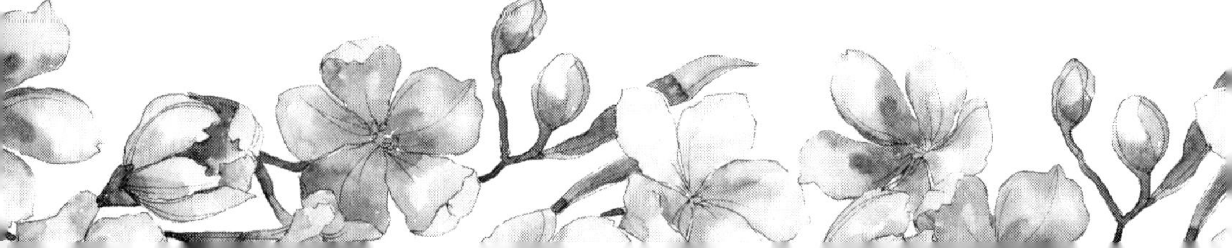

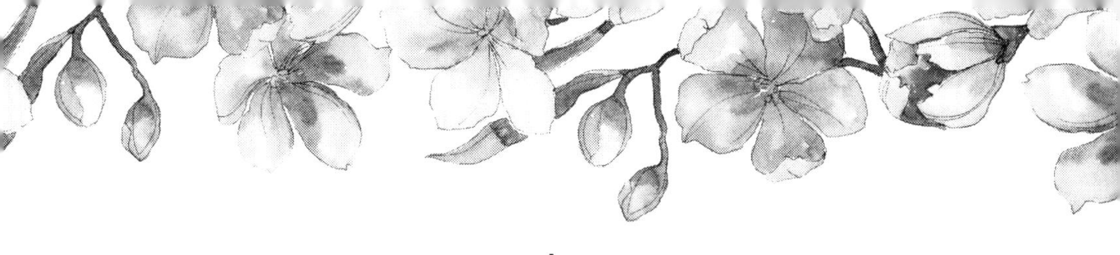

WEEK 5 | RECAP

HOW HAS THIS WEEK BEEN FOR YOU?

IN WHAT WAYS HAVE YOU GROWN?

WHAT COULD YOU DO BETTER NEXT WEEK?

WEEK 6

Coping Strategies & Self-Care

This week you will focus on nurturing your emotional well-being through coping strategies and self-care. You are going to explore a variety of coping mechanisms that are specific to your personal needs and preferences and will provide you with the tools you need to deal with everything that life throws at you. At this point, you will be strongly pushed to put your physical, mental, and emotional well-being first.

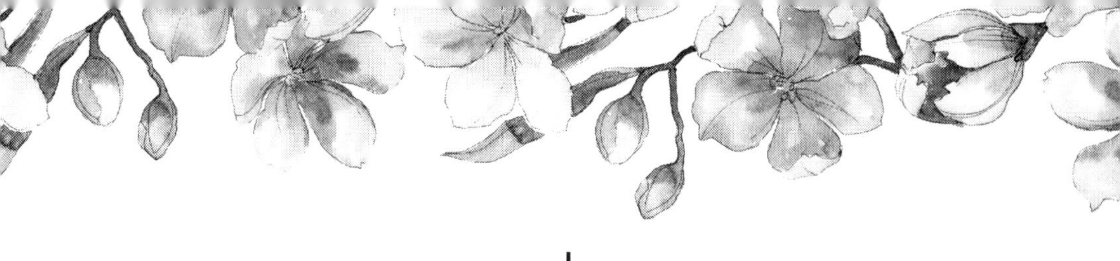

WEEK 6 | DAY 1

HOW DO YOU USUALLY DEAL WITH TOUGH MEMORIES, EMOTIONS OR THOUGHTS?

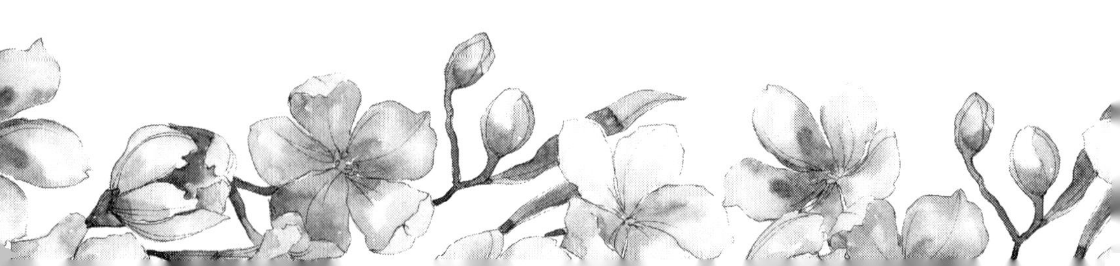

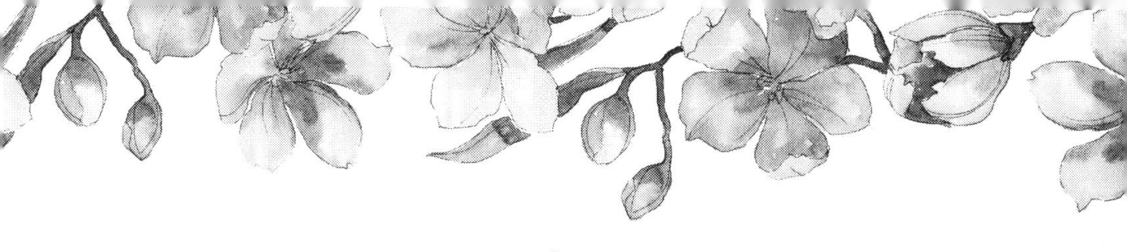

WEEK 6 | DAY 2

WHAT ARE 3 WAYS IN WHICH YOU COULD CULTIVATE A STRONGER SENSE OF SECURITY IN YOUR LIFE?

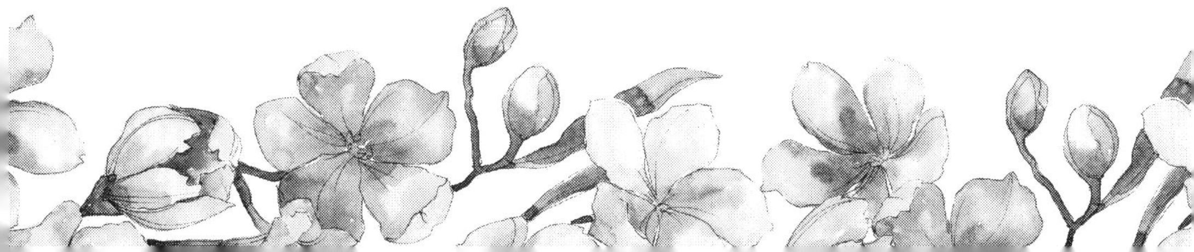

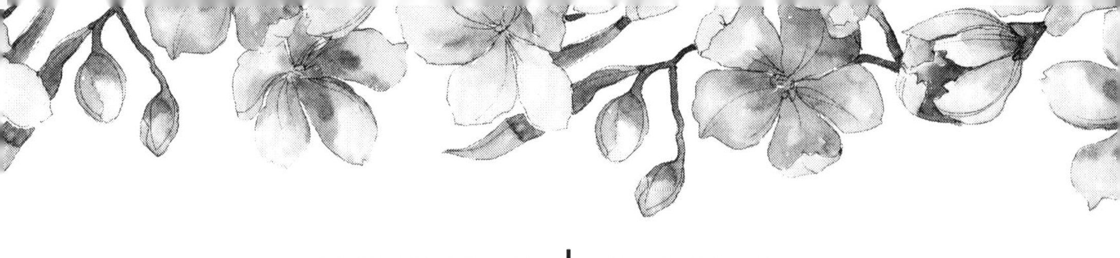

WEEK 6 | DAY 3

HOW DO PHYSICAL HEALTH AND YOUR MENTAL HEALTH CONNECT FOR YOU?

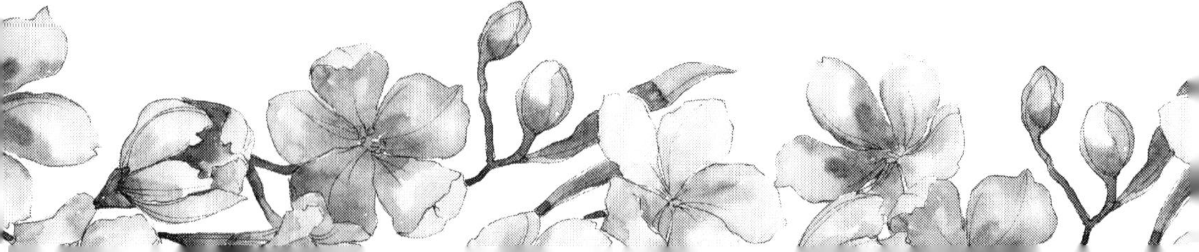

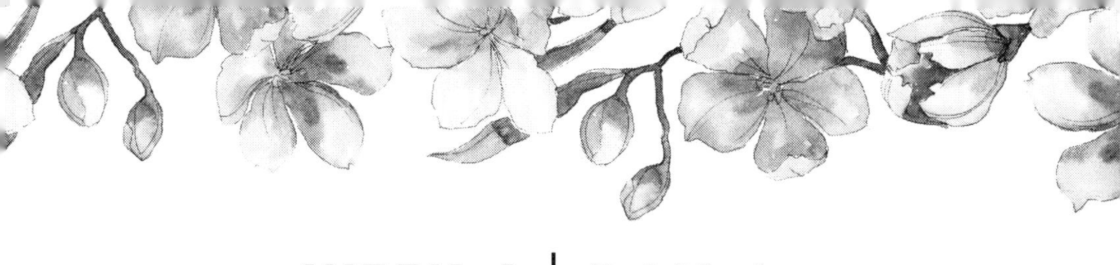

WEEK 6 | DAY 4

WHAT IS A SELF-CARE ACTIVITY THAT BRINGS YOU JOY?

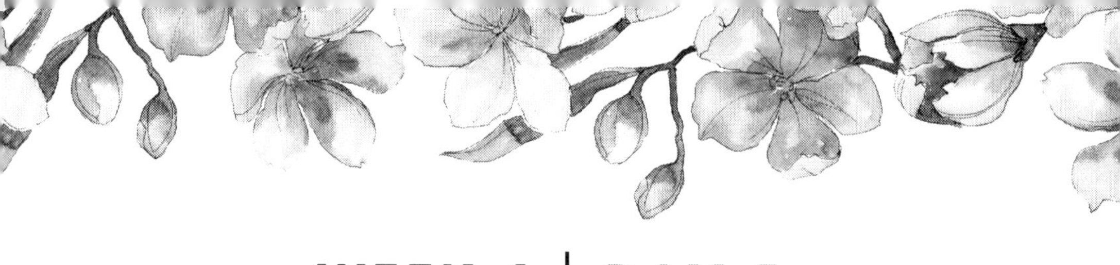

WEEK 6 | DAY 5

WRITE ABOUT A MISTAKE IN YOUR PAST THAT YOU WERE ABLE TO FORGIVE YOURSELF FOR:

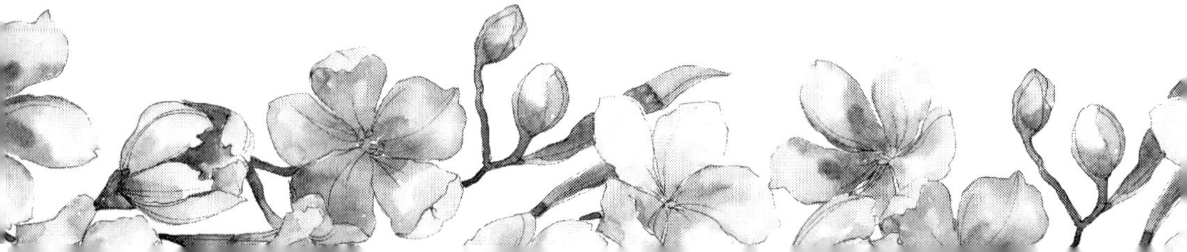

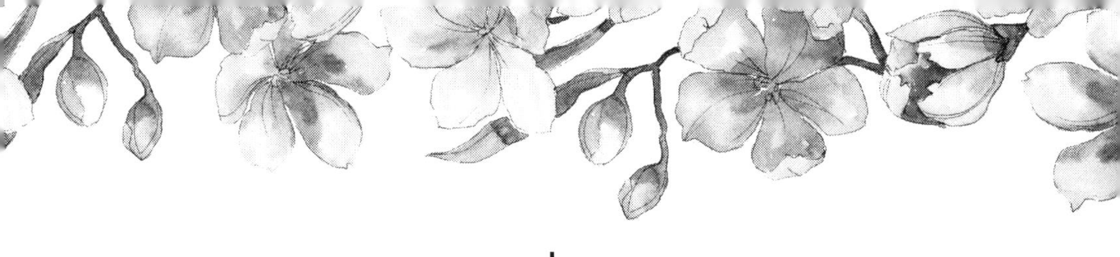

WEEK 6 | DAY 6

HOW CAN YOU STAY MORE PRESENT IN YOUR DAY-TO-DAY LIFE?

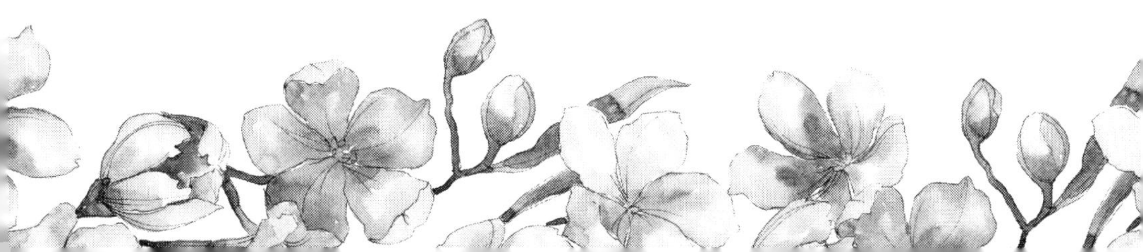

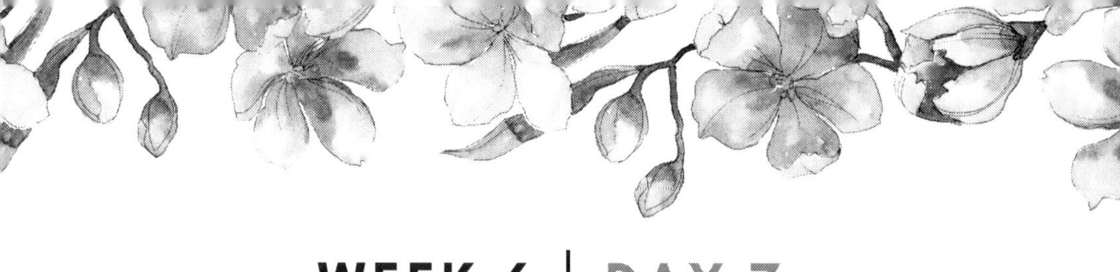

WEEK 6 | DAY 7

RESEARCH AND LIST 3 GROUNDING TECHNIQUES YOU CAN FALL BACK ON IN MOMENTS OF ANXIETY:

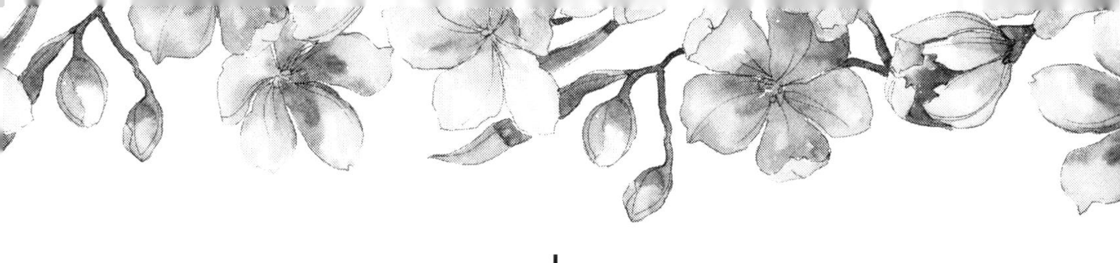

WEEK 6 | RECAP

HOW HAS THIS WEEK BEEN FOR YOU?

IN WHAT WAYS HAVE YOU GROWN?

WHAT COULD YOU DO BETTER NEXT WEEK?

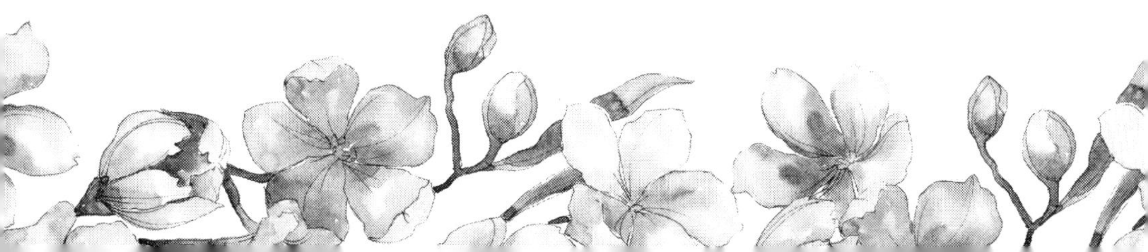

WEEK 7

Processing & Healing

In week seven you will bravely confront the core wounds and emotions that have been buried deep within. You will explore specific experiences and address recurring thoughts that still impact you. Maybe you will encounter some seeming setbacks as you work your way through the layers of healing. Remember to be kind to yourself and embrace the power of resilience as you find methods to go forward.

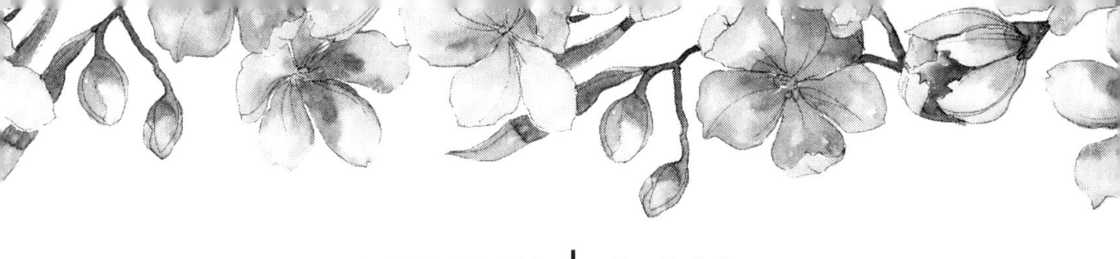

WEEK 7 | DAY 1

ARE THERE ANY RECURRING THOUGHTS YOU HAVE REGARDING YOUR TRAUMA?

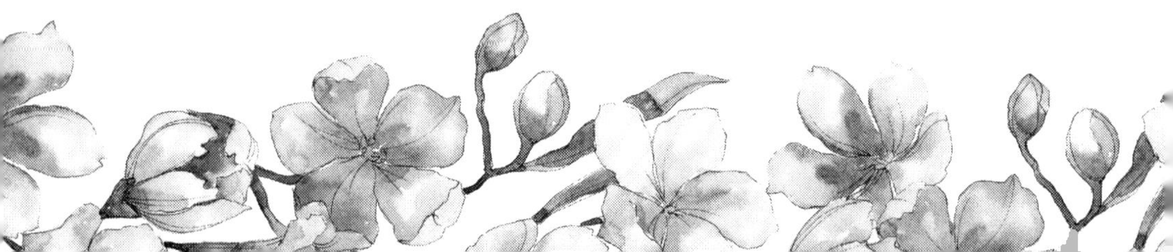

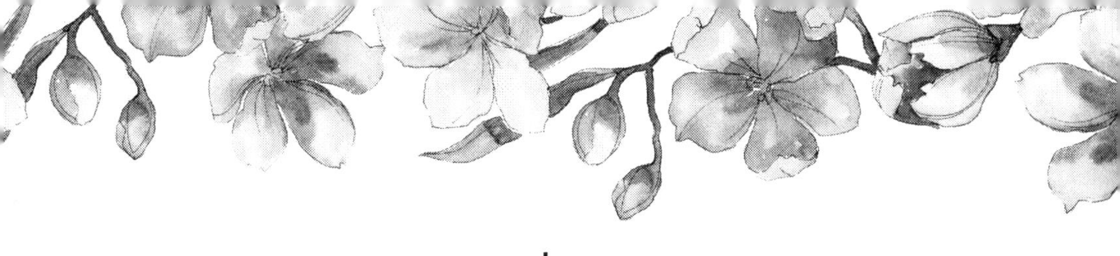

WEEK 7 | DAY 2

DID YOU HAVE ANY SIGNIFICANT REALIZATIONS OR INSIGHTS REGARDING YOUR TRAUMA?

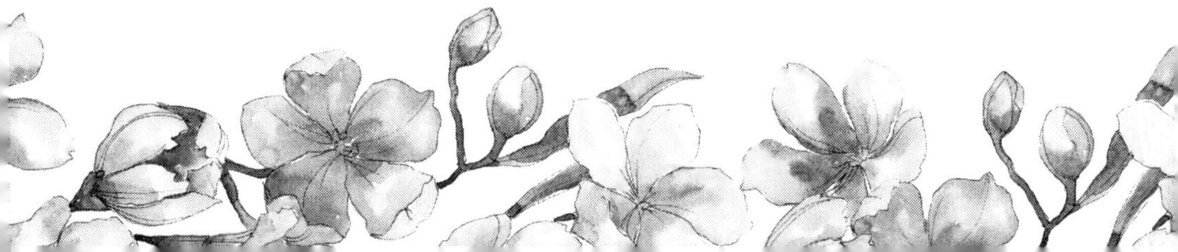

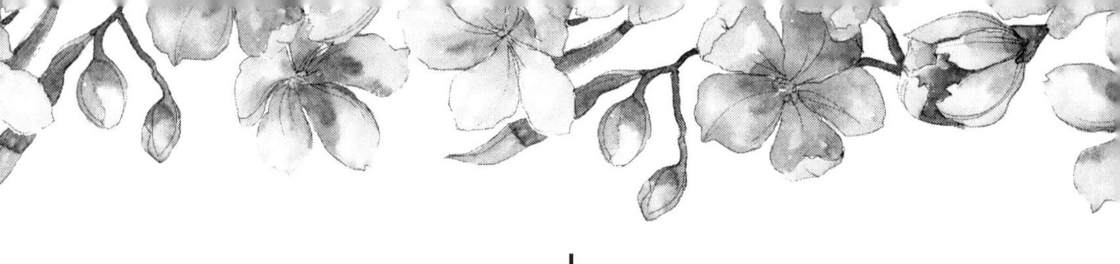

WEEK 7 | DAY 3

HOW HAS TRAUMA IMPACTED YOUR SENSE OF IDENTITY?

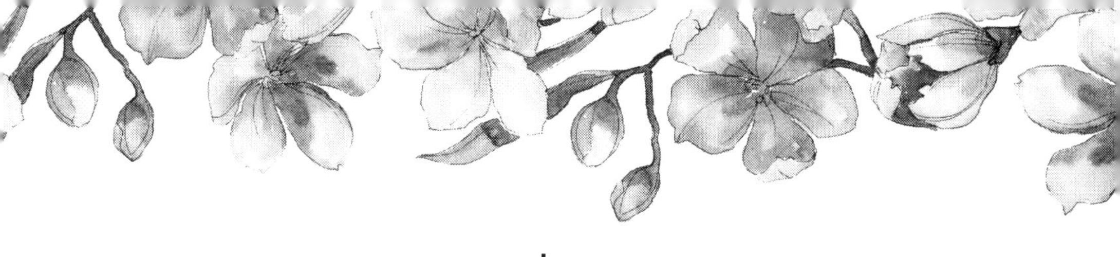

WEEK 7 | DAY 4

HAVE YOU EXPERIENCED ANY SEEMING SETBACKS DURING YOUR HEALING JOURNEY? HOW CAN YOU DEVELOPE MORE RESILIENCE?

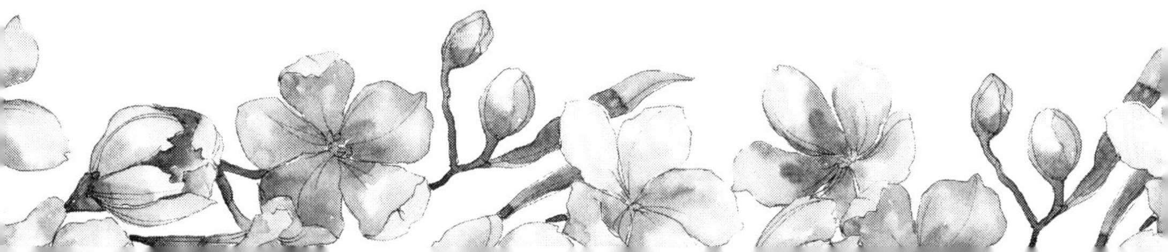

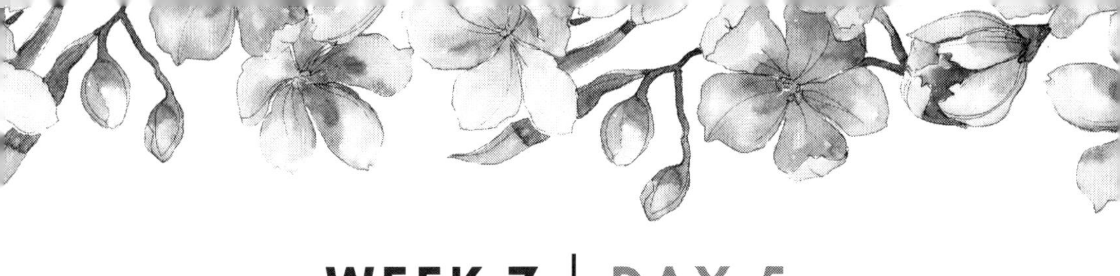

WEEK 7 | DAY 5

DESCRIBE A CHALLENGING EMOTION YOU STILL FIND DIFFICULT TO PROCESS. WHAT CAN YOU DO TO UNDERSTAND THIS EMOTION BETTER?

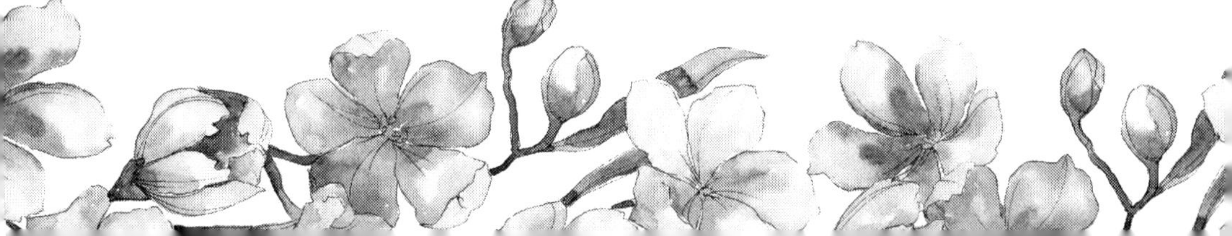

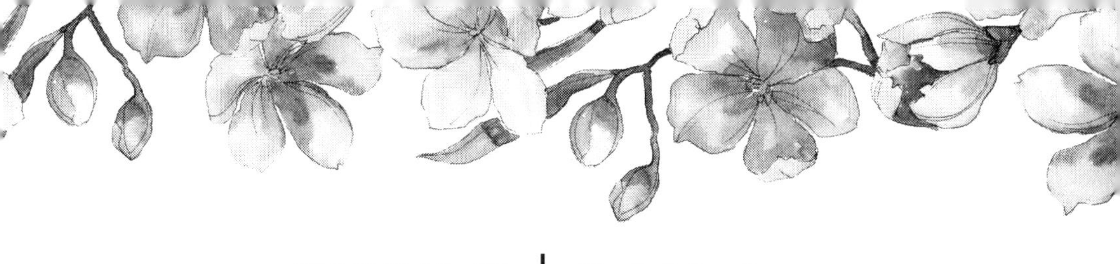

WEEK 7 | DAY 6

WHAT KIND OF SUPPORT DO YOU WISH YOU HAD RECEIVED DURING OR AFTER YOUR TRAUMATIC EXPERIENCE?

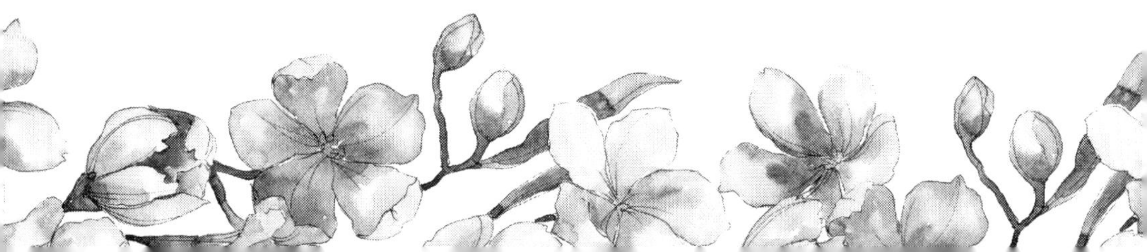

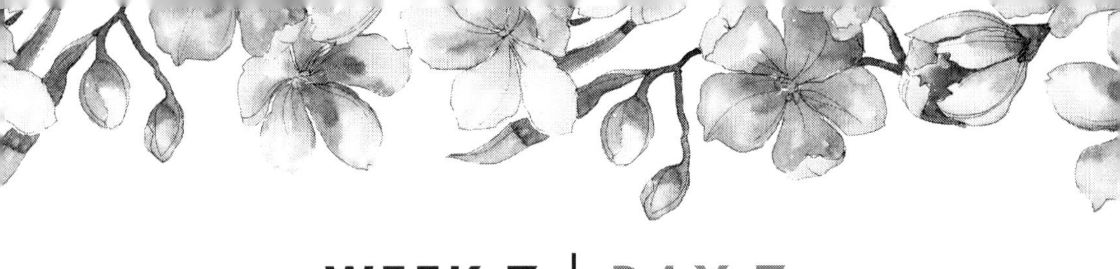

WEEK 7 | DAY 7

DO YOU EVER FEEL LIKE SOCIETY EXPECTS YOU TO JUST BE OK?

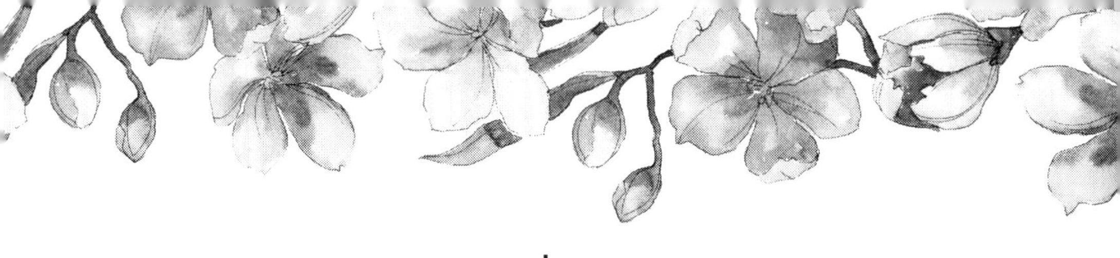

WEEK 7 | RECAP

HOW HAS THIS WEEK BEEN FOR YOU?

IN WHAT WAYS HAVE YOU GROWN?

WHAT COULD YOU DO BETTER NEXT WEEK?

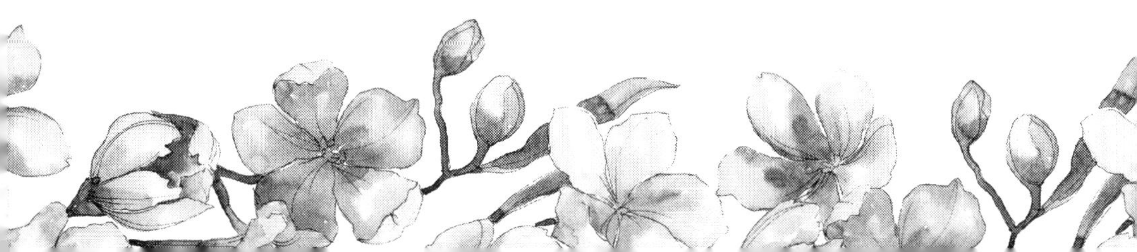

WEEK 8

Reframing Negative Beliefs

In this empowering stage of your trauma healing journey, you will actively engage in reframing negative beliefs that have been rooted in past traumas. You'll discover how certain limiting beliefs have shaped your thoughts, emotions, and actions and challenge the ones that have kept you from reaching your full potential until now. Benefit from this opportunity to take on a more positive and hopeful perspective and improve your state of mind.

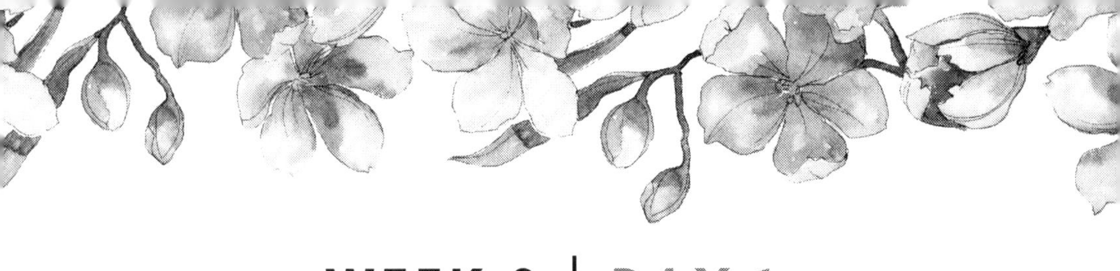

WEEK 8 | DAY 1

DO YOU HOLD ANY NEGATIVE BELIEFS THAT YOU KNOW TO BE FALSE?

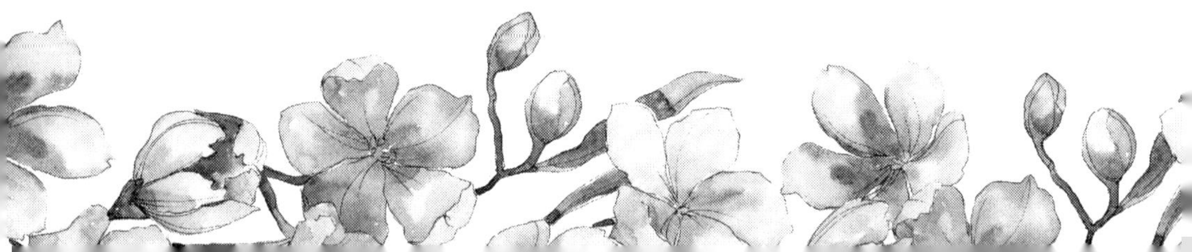

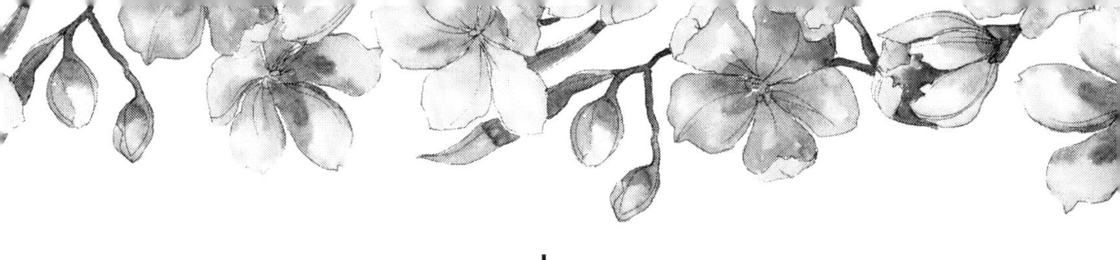

WEEK 8 | DAY 2

DO YOU EVER FEEL A SENSE OF PERFECTIONISM? CAN THAT HOLD YOU BACK SOMETIMES?

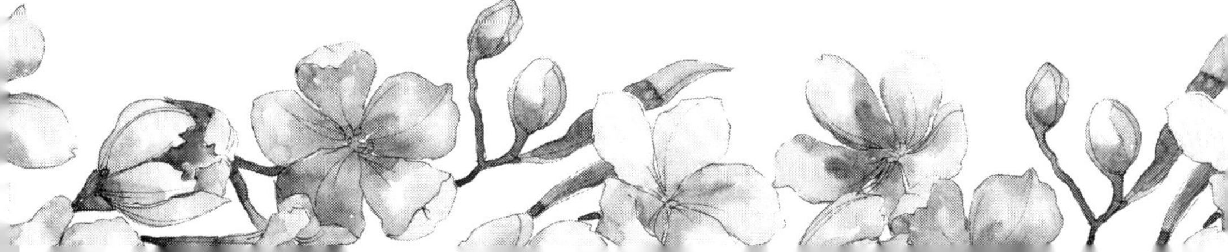

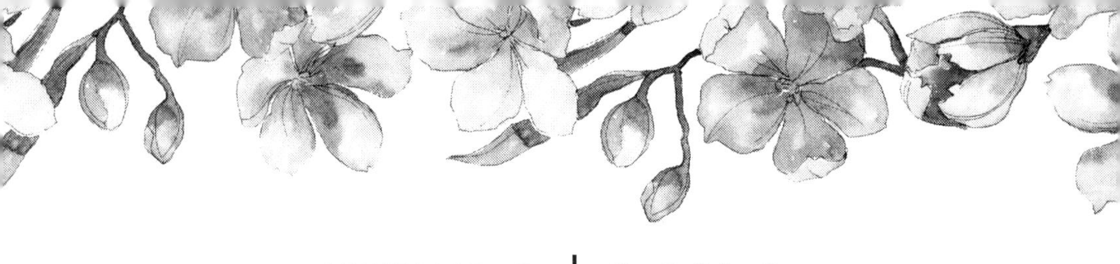

WEEK 8 | DAY 3

HOW HAS YOUR TRAUMA IMPACTED YOUR SENSE OF SELF-WORTH?

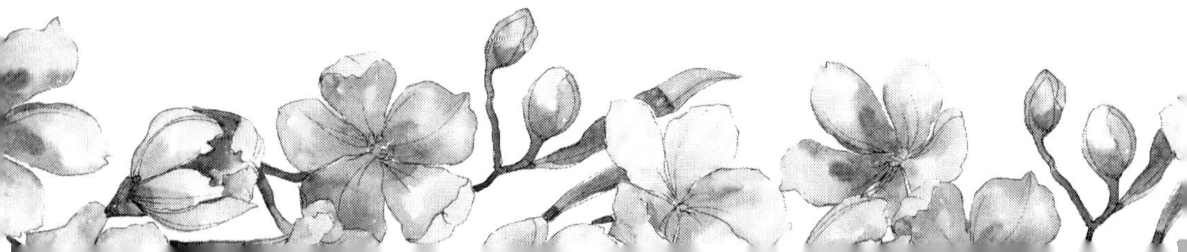

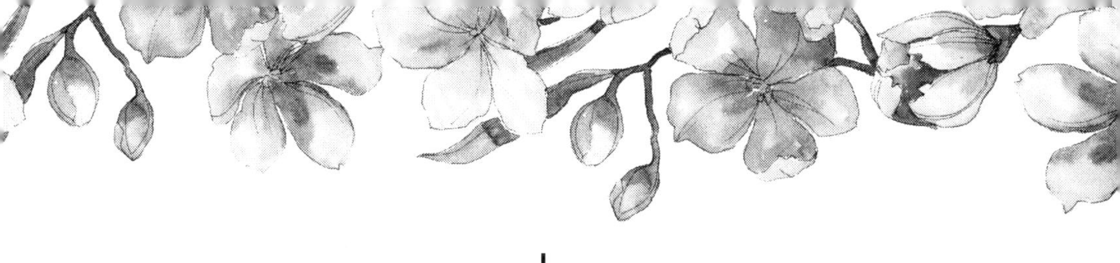

WEEK 8 | DAY 4

HAS ANYTHING ABOUT YOUR VIEW OF THE WORLD CHANGED SINCE YOU WENT THROUGH TRAUMA?

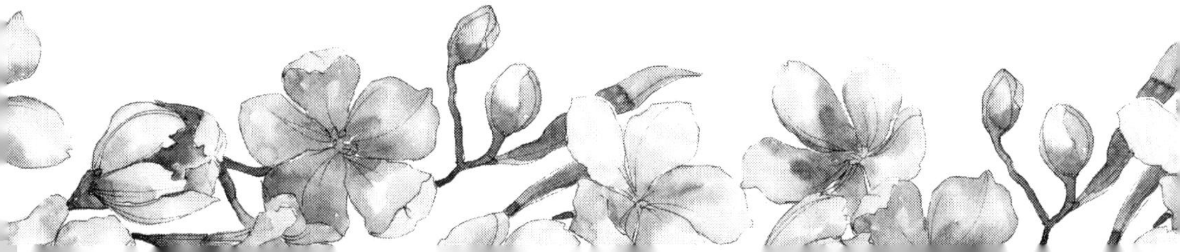

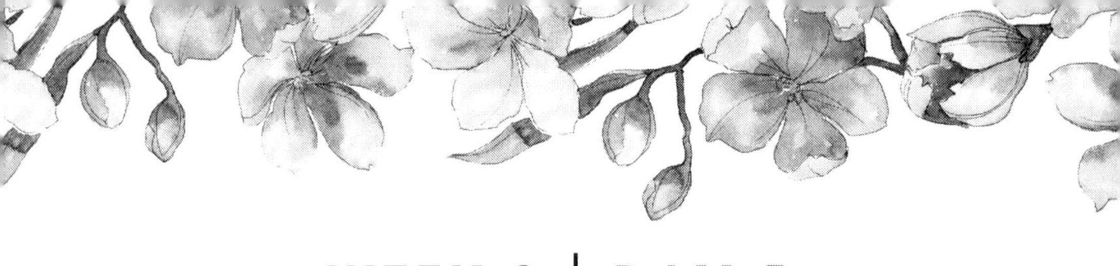

WEEK 8 | DAY 5

IDENTIFY A NEGATIVE BELIEF YOU HOLD ABOUT YOURSELF. CAN YOU FIGURE OUT WHERE IT ORIGINATED?

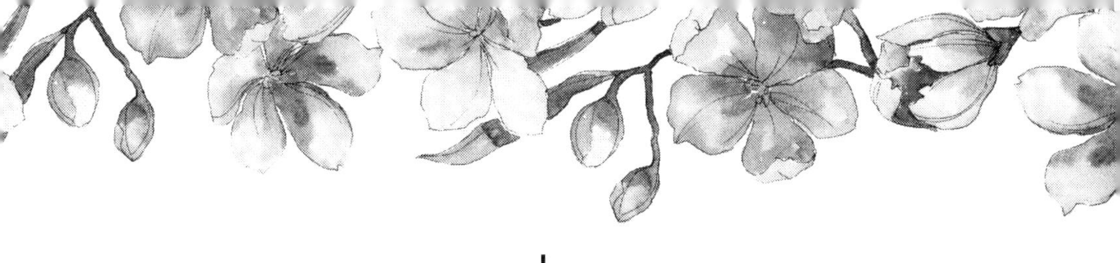

WEEK 8 | DAY 6

DO YOU HAVE ANY LIMITING BELIEFS ABOUT YOUR ABILITY TO MOVE ON FROM THIS?

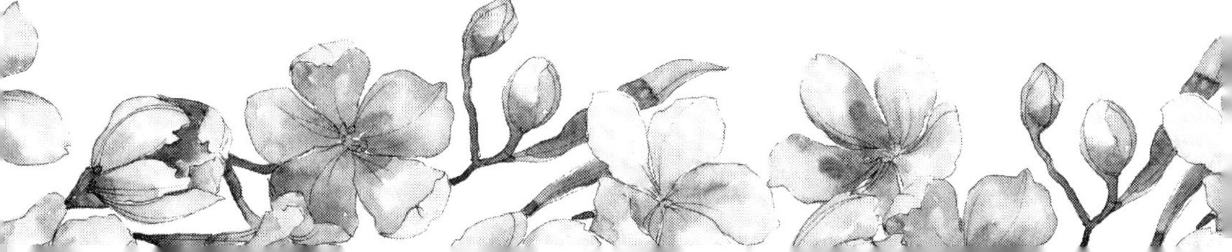

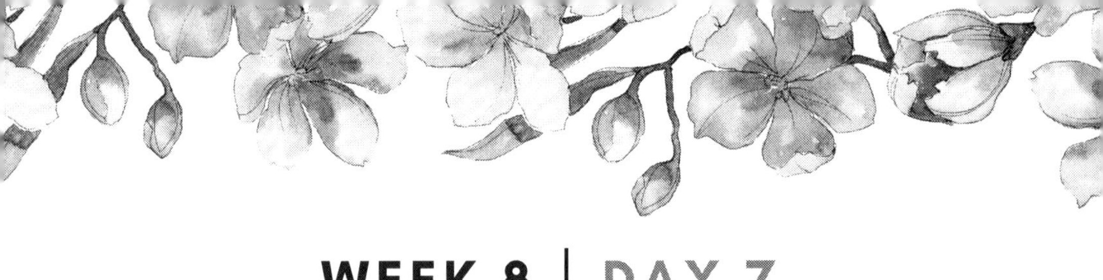

WEEK 8 | DAY 7

LIST 3 MAJOR FEARS THAT COME UP AS A RESULT OF YOUR NEGATIVE BELIEF, THEN WRITE DOWN 3 POSITIVE AFFIRMATIONS THAT COUNTER THEM:

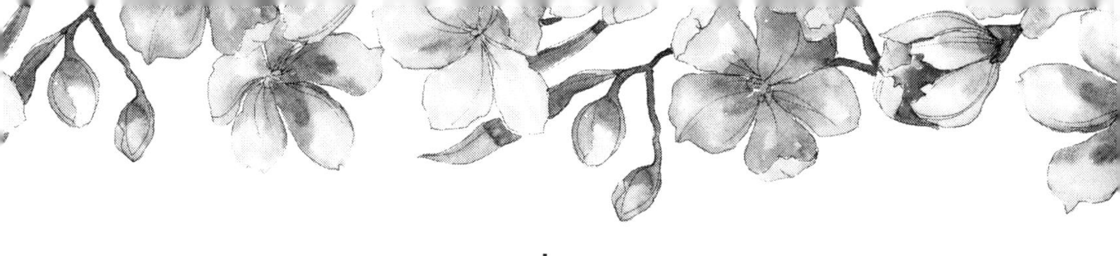

WEEK 8 | RECAP

HOW HAS THIS WEEK BEEN FOR YOU?

IN WHAT WAYS HAVE YOU GROWN?

WHAT COULD YOU DO BETTER NEXT WEEK?

WEEK 9

Forgiveness & Self-Compassion

This week you will explore the power of forgiving others and, most importantly, yourself. You will confront lingering feelings of resentment and liberate yourself from the burden of holding onto the past. Take advantage of the chance to be nice to yourself this week as you treat your inner self with compassion and understanding. As you cultivate forgiveness and self-compassion, you will allow yourself to heal from within and emotionally free yourself.

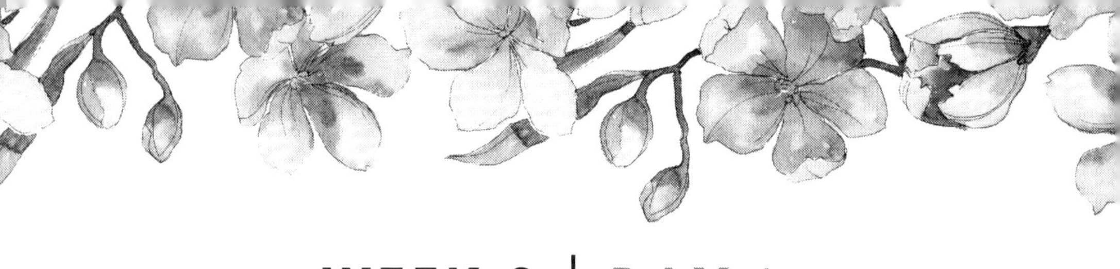

WEEK 9 | DAY 1

WHAT DOES FORGIVENESS MEAN TO YOU?

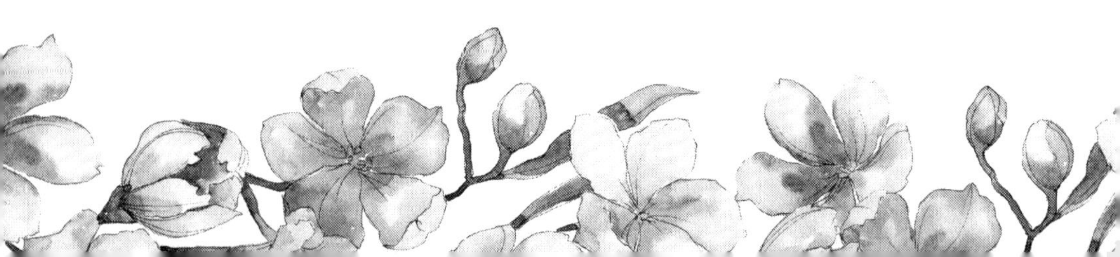

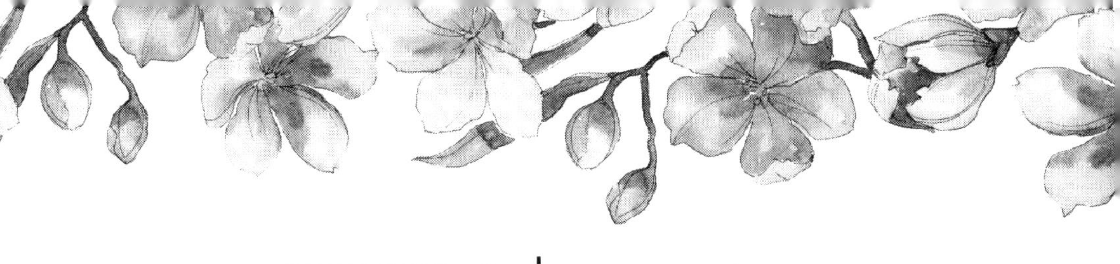

WEEK 9 | DAY 2

WRITE A LETTER TO SOMEONE WHO HAS HURT YOU, EXPRESSING YOUR FEELINGS (IT'S JUST FOR YOU, NO NEED TO SEND IT):

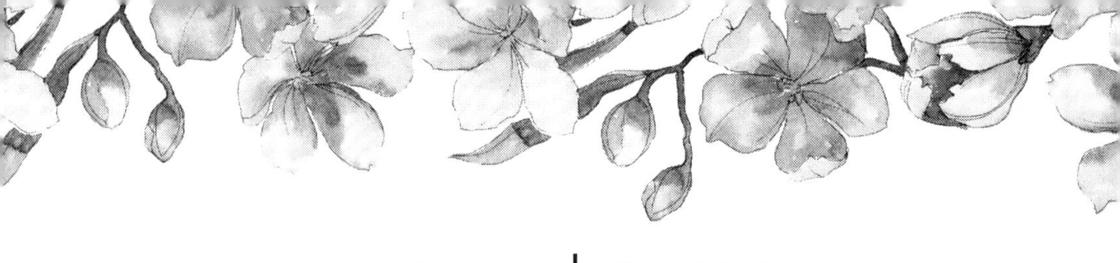

WEEK 9 | DAY 3

CAN IT SOMETIMES BE CHALLENGING FOR YOU TO ACCEPT LOVE AND SUPPORT FROM OTHERS? WHY?

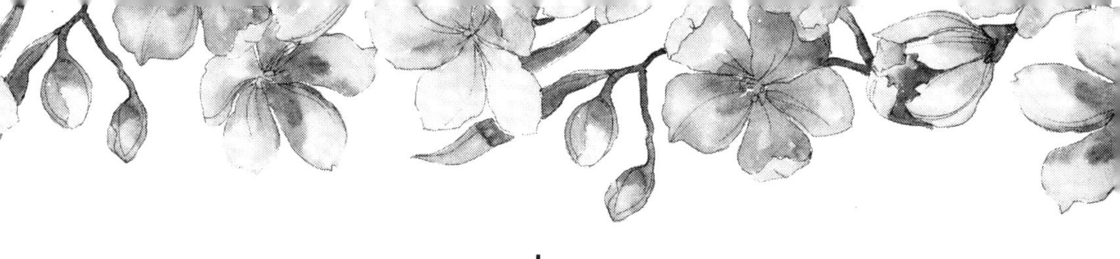

WEEK 9 | DAY 4

HOW DOES THE CONCEPT OF "LETTING GO" FIT INTO YOUR HEALING JOURNEY?

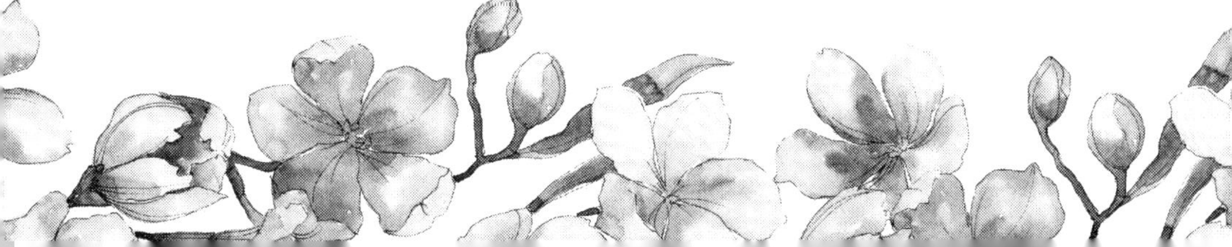

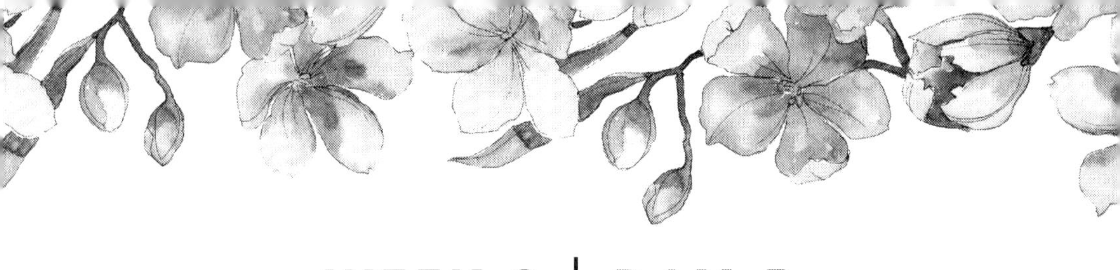

WEEK 9 | DAY 5

WHEN WAS THE LAST TIME YOU TRULY FORGAVE YOURSELF FOR A MISTAKE YOU MADE?

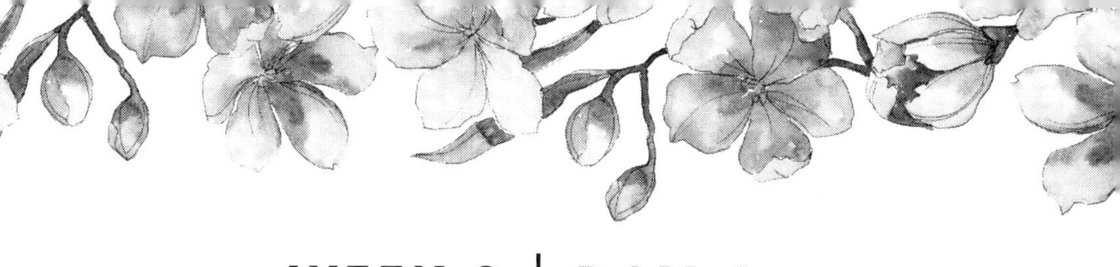

WEEK 9 | DAY 6

DO YOU STRUGGLE WITH SHOWING YOURSELF COMPASSION? HOW DOES THAT MAKE YOU FEEL?

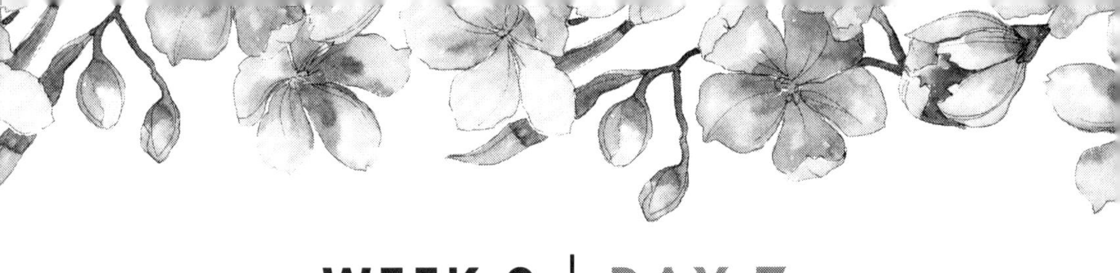

WEEK 9 | DAY 7

IN WHAT WAYS CAN YOU BE MORE COMPASSIONATE AND KIND WITH YOURSELF MOVING FORWARD?

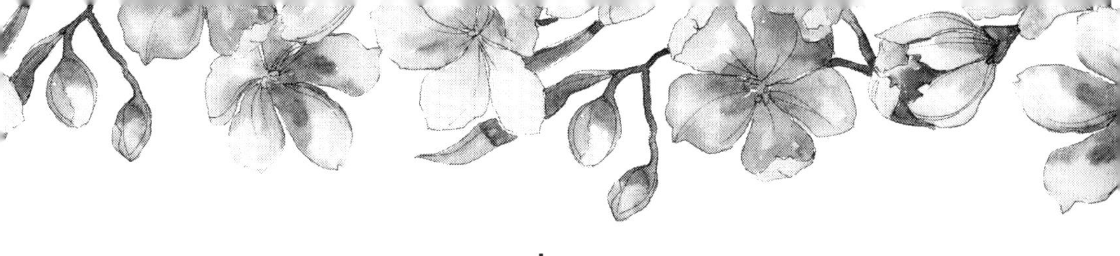

WEEK 9 | RECAP

HOW HAS THIS WEEK BEEN FOR YOU?

IN WHAT WAYS HAVE YOU GROWN?

WHAT COULD YOU DO BETTER NEXT WEEK?

WEEK 10

Growth & Resilience

This week is all about celebrating your resilience and perseverance during your transformational journey. You will reflect on how your trauma has made you stronger, and look back on moments when you have compromised your boundaries to satisfy others. By learning from those experiences you can start to nurture healthier boundaries and protect your well-being. With hope and self-empowerment guiding you, you can look towards the future with confidence, knowing you are continuously evolving and growing.

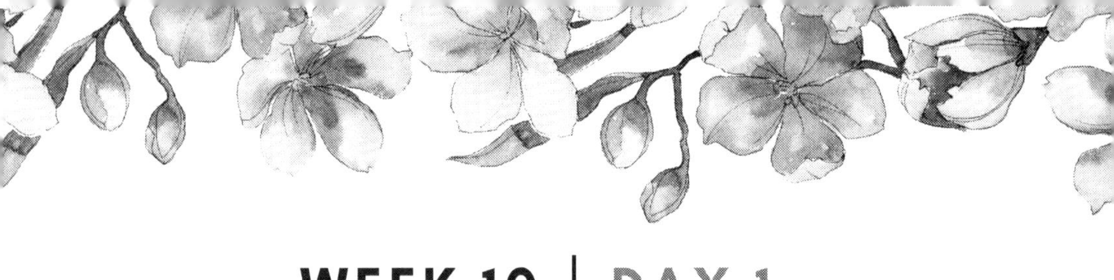

WEEK 10 | DAY 1

IS THERE A WAY IN WHICH YOUR TRAUMA HAS MADE YOU STRONGER?

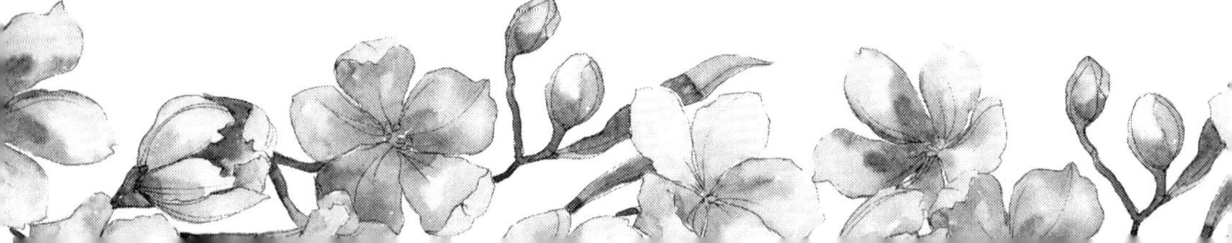

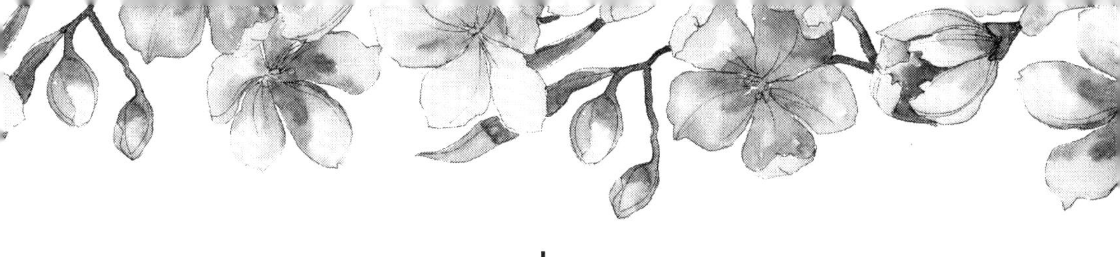

WEEK 10 | DAY 2

HAVE YOU EVER COMPROMISED YOUR OWN BOUNDARIES TO PLEASE OTHERS? HOW DID THAT MAKE YOU FEEL?

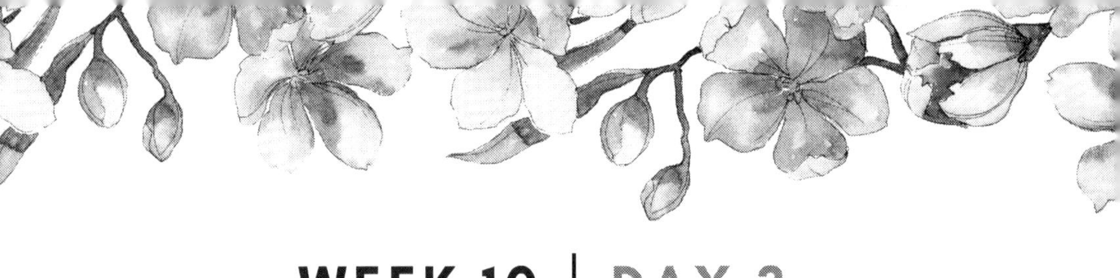

WEEK 10 | DAY 3

WRITE ABOUT A SITUATION WHERE YOU SUCCESSFULLY SET BOUNDARIES TO PROTECT YOUR WELL-BEING. HOW CAN YOU DO MORE OF THAT IN THE FUTURE?

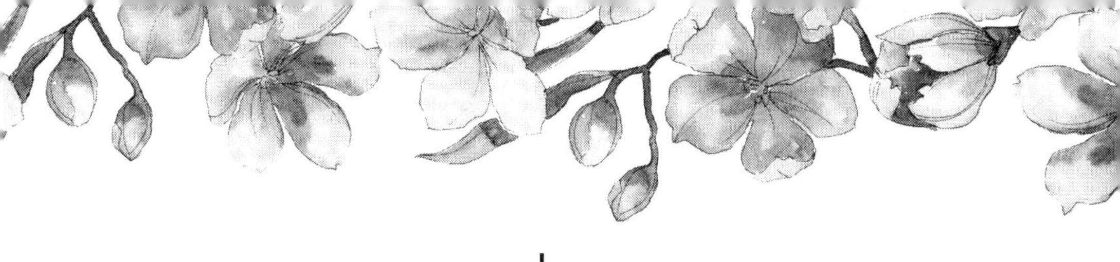

WEEK 10 | DAY 4

WAS THERE EVER A SITUATION WHERE YOU WERE SURPRISED BY YOUR OWN STRENGTH?

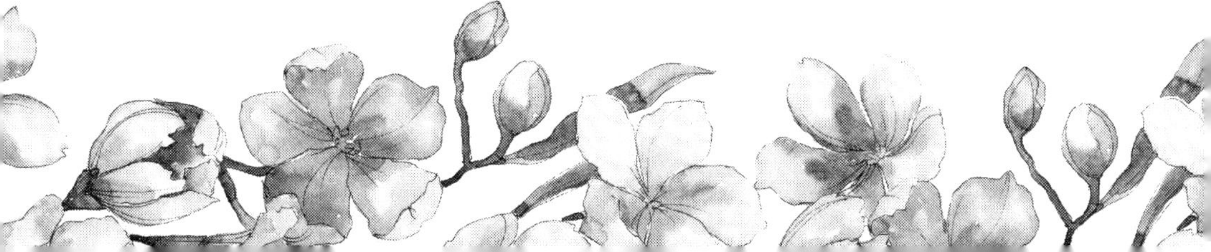

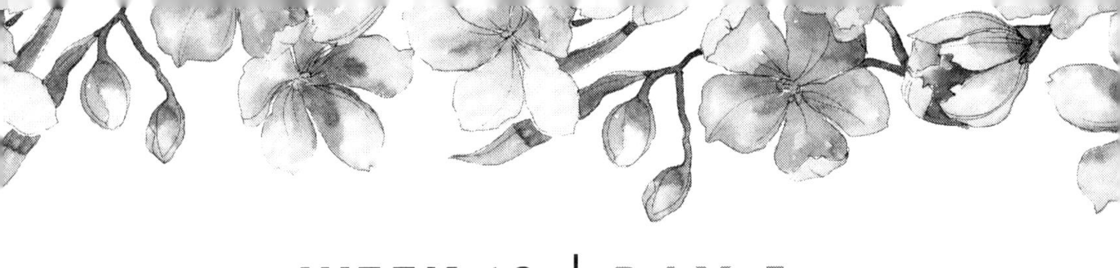

WEEK 10 | DAY 5

WHAT ARE THE 3 QUALITIES THAT YOU ADMIRE THE MOST IN YOURSELF?

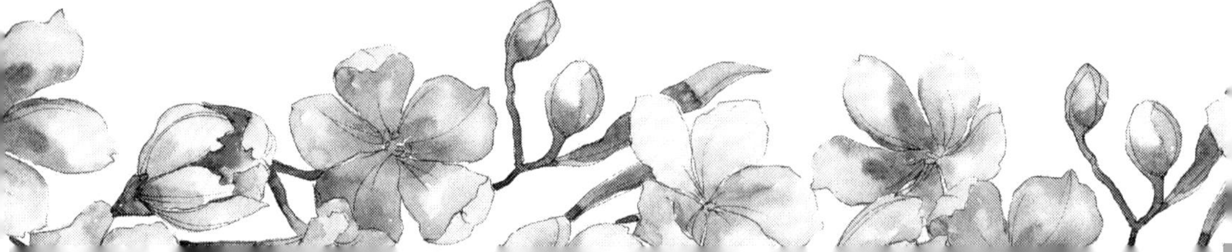

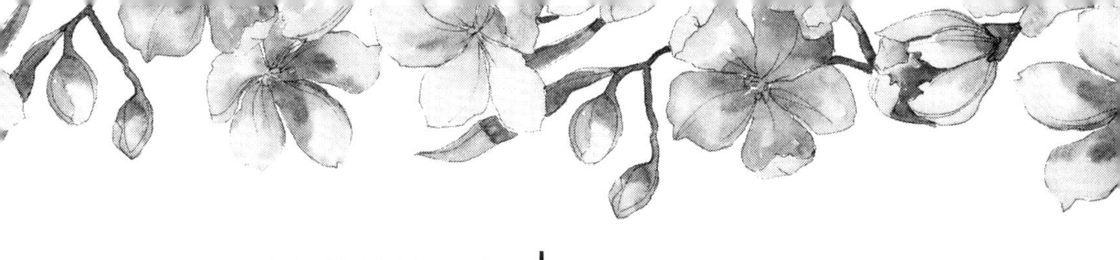

WEEK 10 | DAY 6

IN WHAT WAYS HAVE YOU EXPERIENCED PERSONAL GROWTH SINCE STARTING YOUR HEALING JOURNEY?

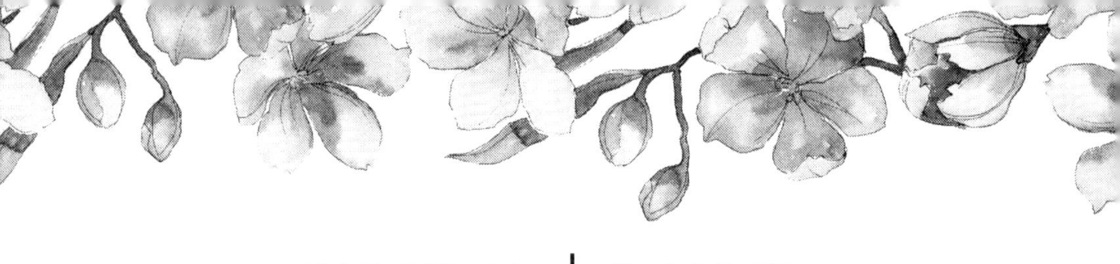

WEEK 10 | DAY 7

WRITE A LETTER TO YOUR YOUNGER SELF. HOW WOULD YOU SUPPORT HER AS THE PERSON YOU ARE NOW?

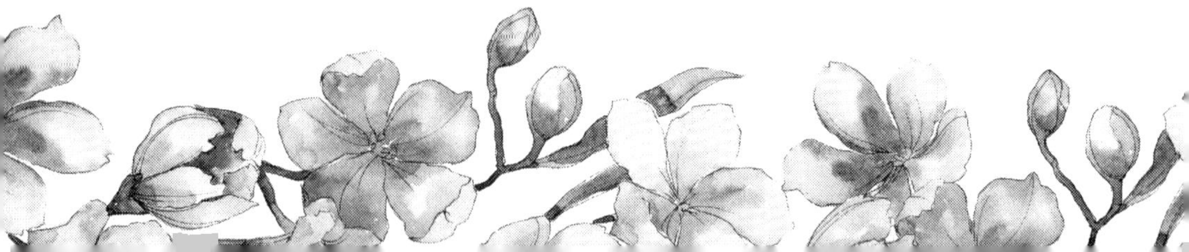

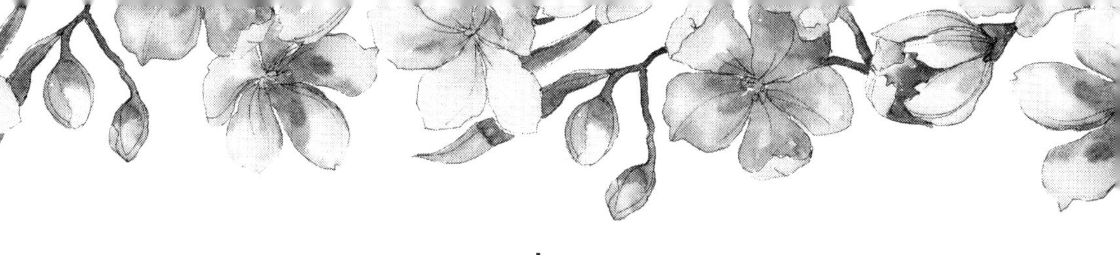

WEEK 10 | RECAP

HOW HAS THIS WEEK BEEN FOR YOU?

IN WHAT WAYS HAVE YOU GROWN?

WHAT COULD YOU DO BETTER NEXT WEEK?

WEEK 11

Building Supportive Relationships

In week eleven you will reflect on the impact your trauma has had on your relationships with the people in your life and explore the connections that uplift and empower you. Through nurturing and cultivating positive relationships you build a support system that can foster growth, trust, and genuine connection, making your journey all the more enjoyable and much less difficult.

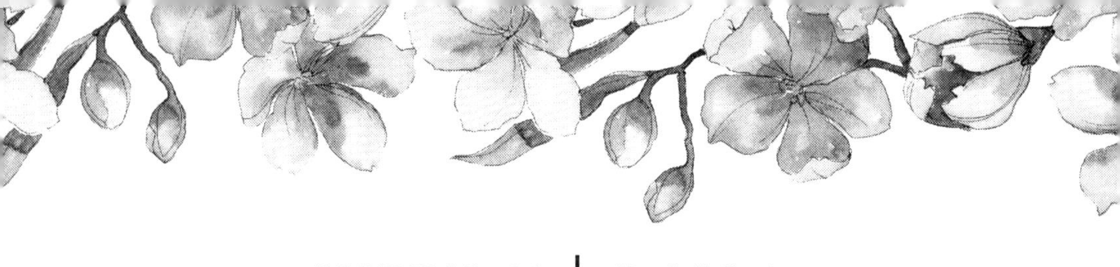

WEEK 11 | DAY 1

HOW DOES YOUR EXPERIENCE IMPACT THE CURRENT RELATIONSHIPS IN YOUR LIFE?

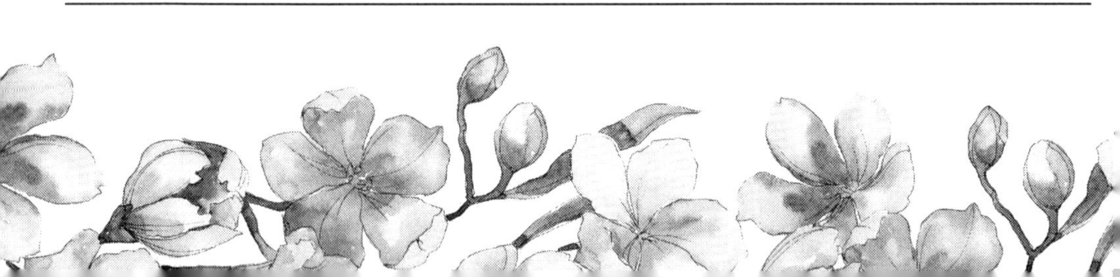

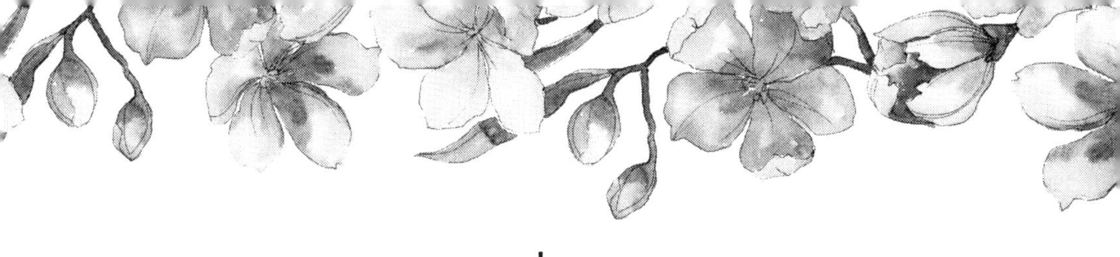

WEEK 11 | DAY 2

WHO OR WHAT HAS BEEN PARTICULARLY SUPPORTIVE DURING YOUR HEALING JOURNEY?

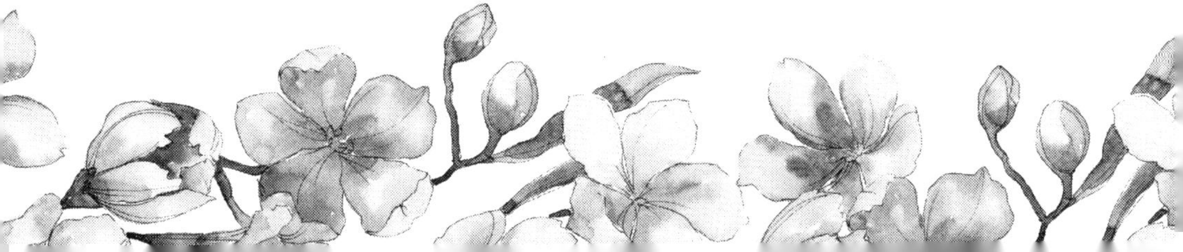

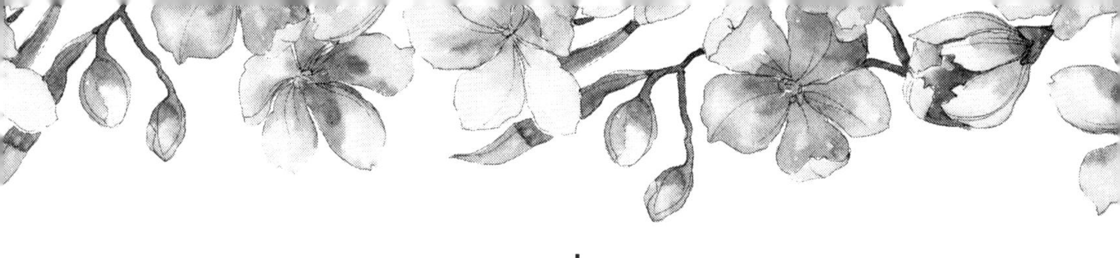

WEEK 11 | DAY 3

HOW HAS YOUR TRAUMA AFFECTED YOUR ABILITY TO TRUST OTHER PEOPLE?

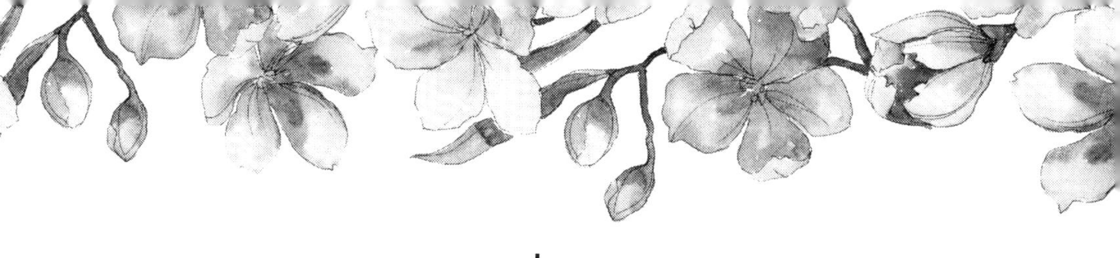

WEEK 11 | DAY 4

WRITE ABOUT A TIME WHEN YOU FELT VULNERABLE BUT ALLOWED YOURSELF TO SEEK HELP OR SUPPORT:

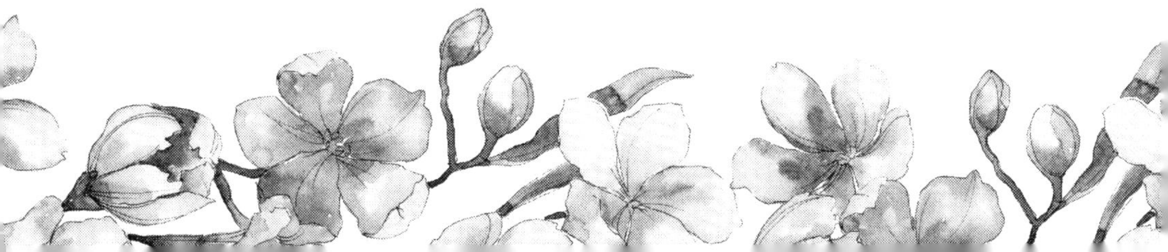

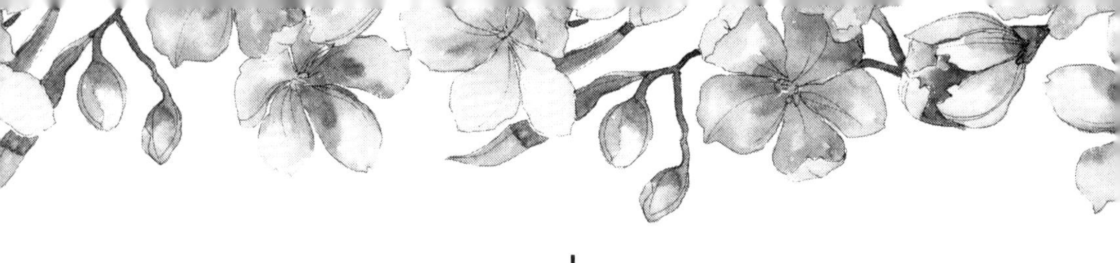

WEEK 11 | DAY 5

WRITE ABOUT 3 POSITIVE ROLE MODELS THAT HAVE INSPIRED AND MOTIVATED YOU:

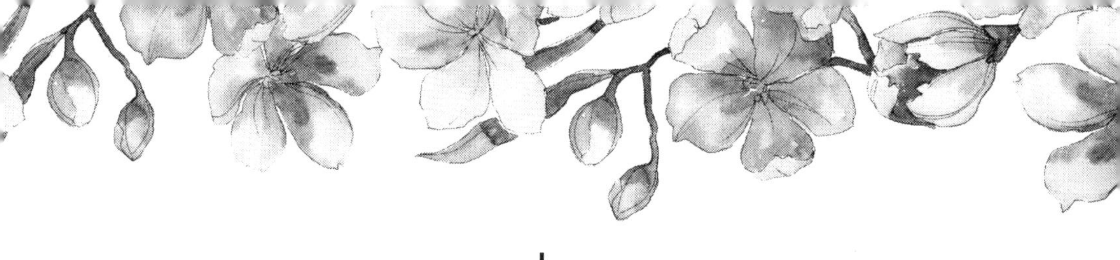

WEEK 11 | DAY 6

WHAT DOES YOUR IDEAL SUPPORT SYSTEM LOOK LIKE?

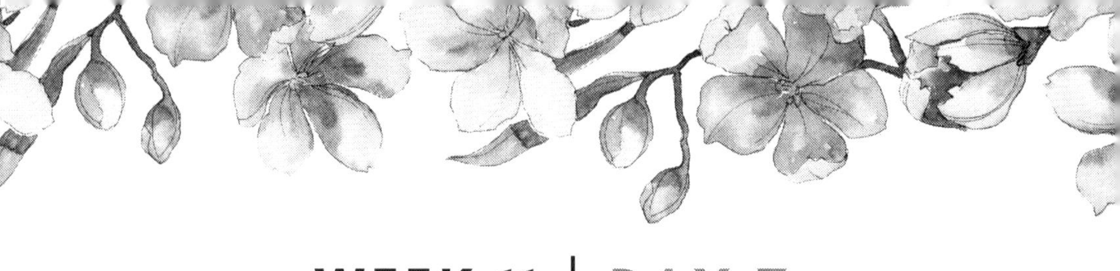

WEEK 11 | DAY 7

ARE THERE WAYS IN WHICH YOU CAN HELP OTHER PEOPLE WHO MAY HAVE GONE THROUGH SOMETHING SIMILAR?

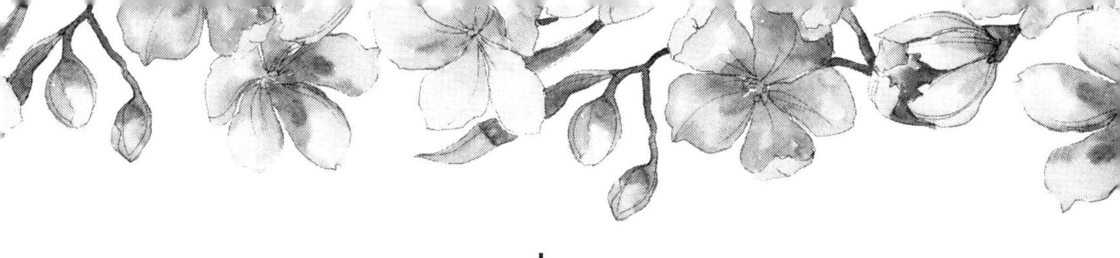

WEEK 11 | RECAP

HOW HAS THIS WEEK BEEN FOR YOU?

IN WHAT WAYS HAVE YOU GROWN?

WHAT COULD YOU DO BETTER NEXT WEEK?

WEEK 12

Reflecting & Moving Forward

In this empowering final stage of your trauma healing journal, you will embark on a journey of profound reflection and forward momentum. You will look back on this 12-week process with a sense of accomplishment, and acknowledge the inner transformation you have gone through. You can be immensely proud of yourself for going through this process and showing up for yourself. Celebrate the milestones and breakthroughs you've experienced during your healing journey and set intentions for the future, envisioning the person you aspire to become and the life you desire.

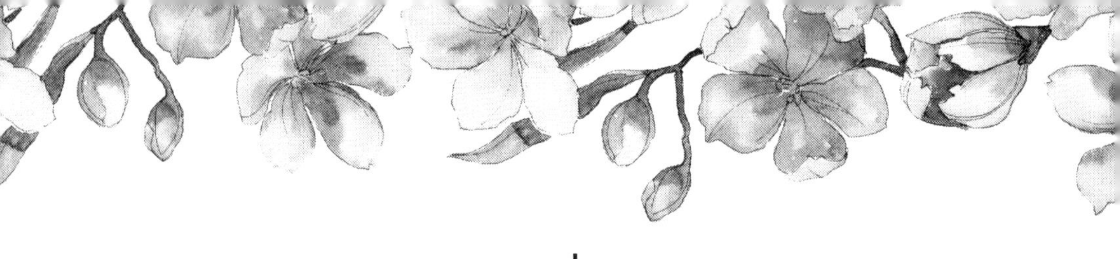

WEEK 12 | DAY 1

REFLECT ON THE PROGRESS YOU HAVE MADE DURING YOUR HEALING JOURNEY:

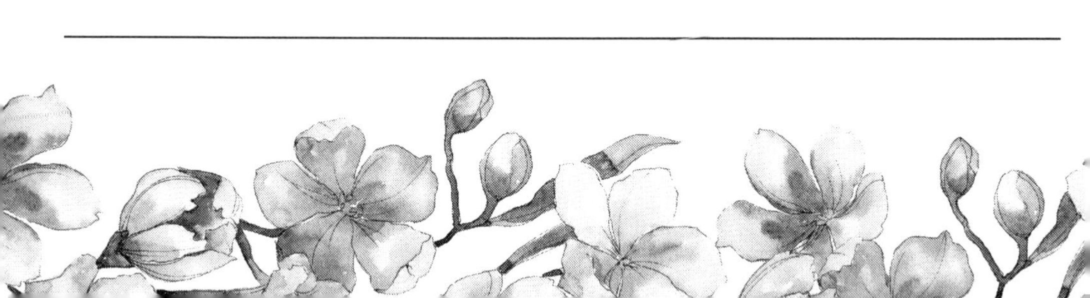

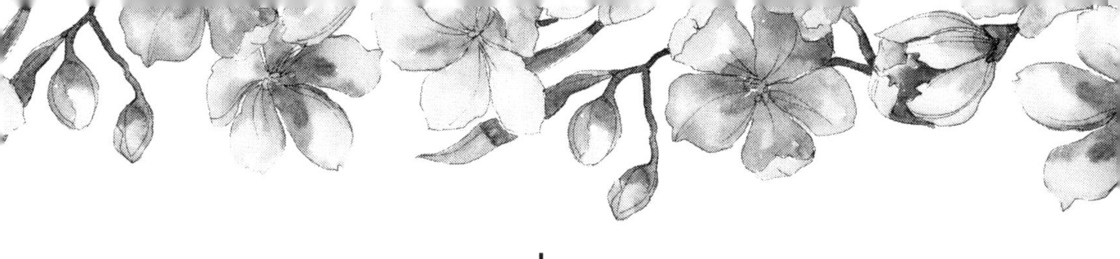

WEEK 12 | DAY 2

WHAT WAS A MOMENT OF UNEXPECTED JOY IN YOUR HEALING JOURNEY?

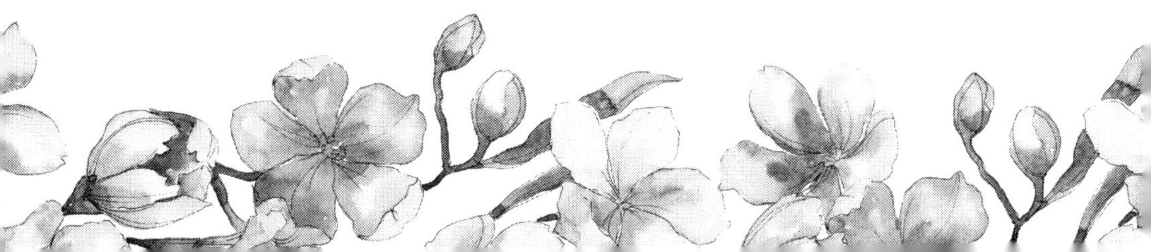

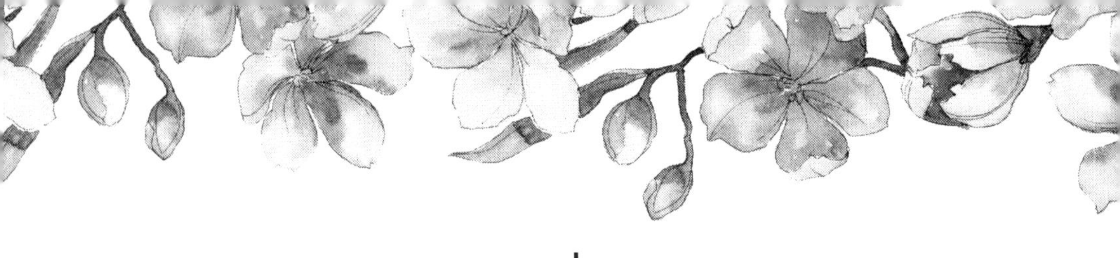

WEEK 12 | DAY 3

WHAT ASPECTS OF YOUR LIFE HAVE IMPROVED SINCE YOU STARTED TO HEAL?

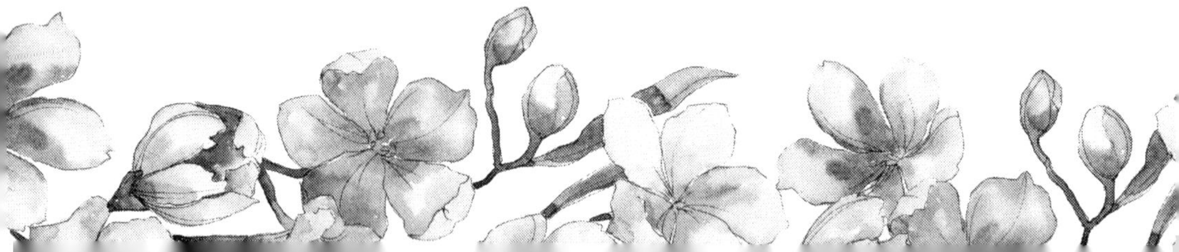

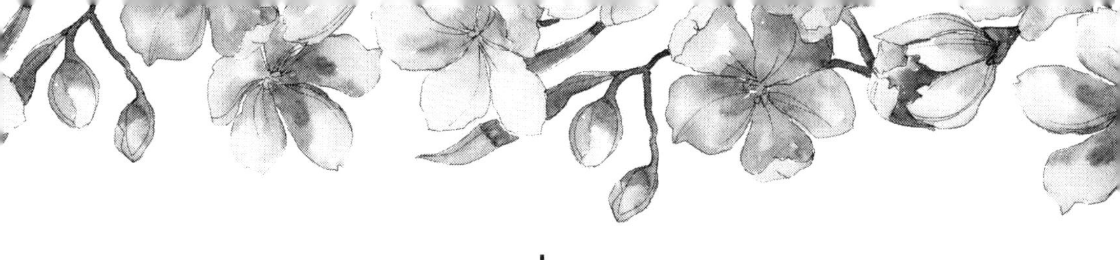

WEEK 12 | DAY 4

WHAT ARE 10 THINGS YOU ARE GRATEFUL FOR IN YOUR LIFE RIGHT NOW?

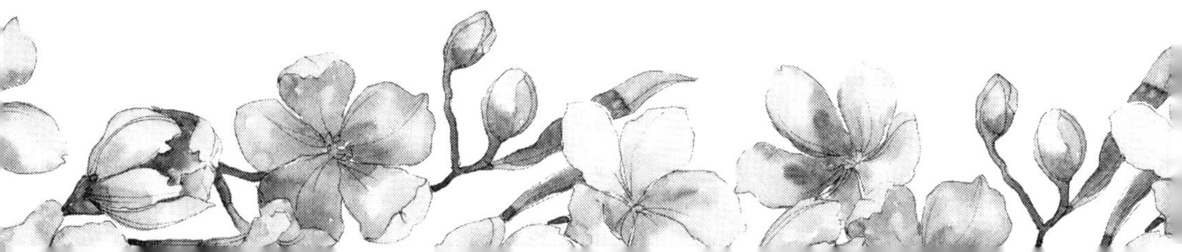

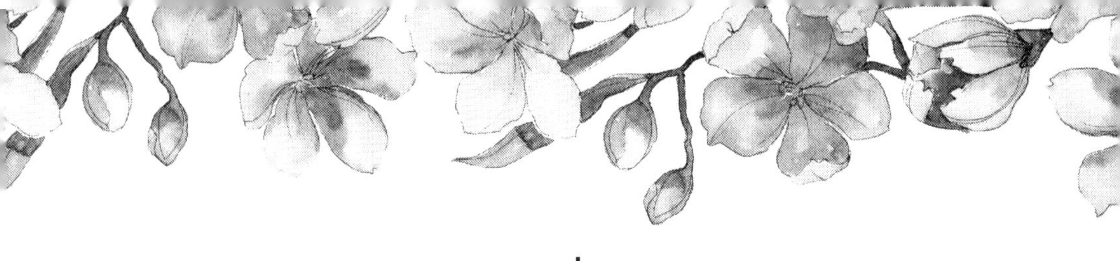

WEEK 12 | DAY 5

HOW CAN YOU REWARD YOURSELF MORE FOR THE PROGRESS YOU ARE MAKING?

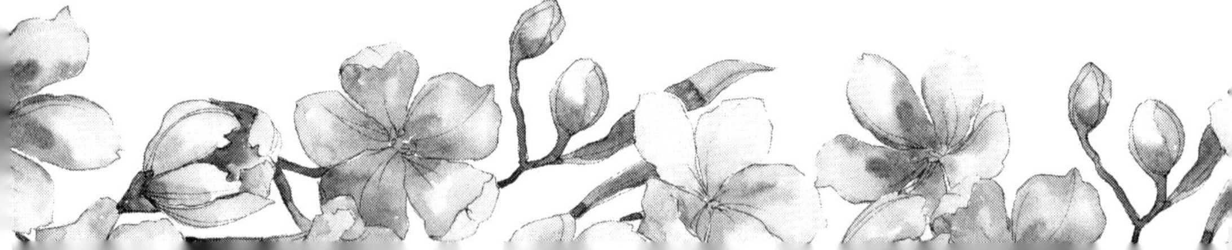

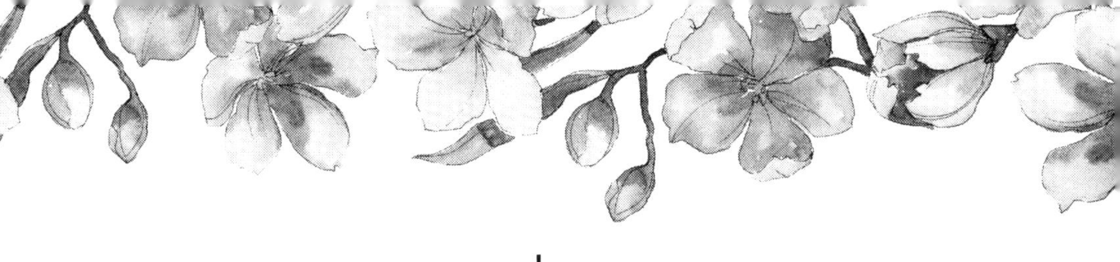

WEEK 12 | DAY 6

WHAT IS YOUR IDEA OF AUTHENTICITY AS YOU MOVE FORWARD IN LIFE?

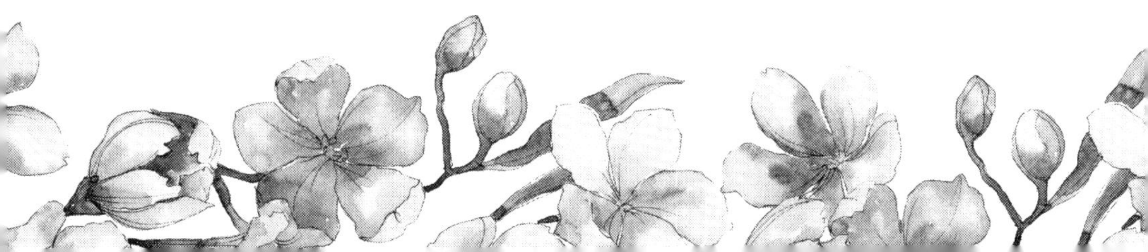

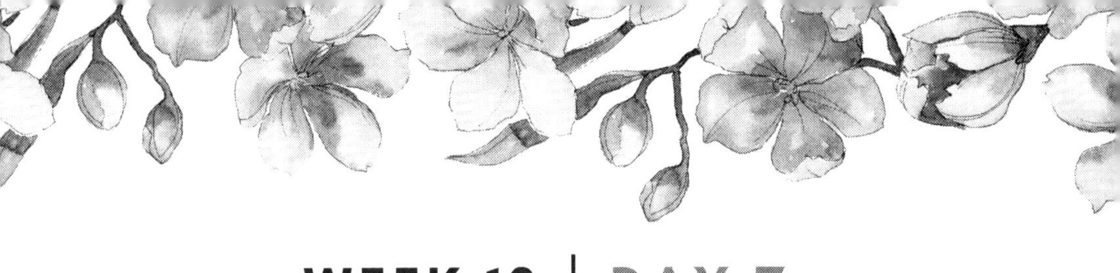

WEEK 12 | DAY 7

WRITE ABOUT A VISION OF YOUR LIFE FILLED WITH HOPE AND POSSIBILITIES. WHO DO YOU SEE YOURSELF BEING? HOW DOES IT MAKE YOU FEEL?

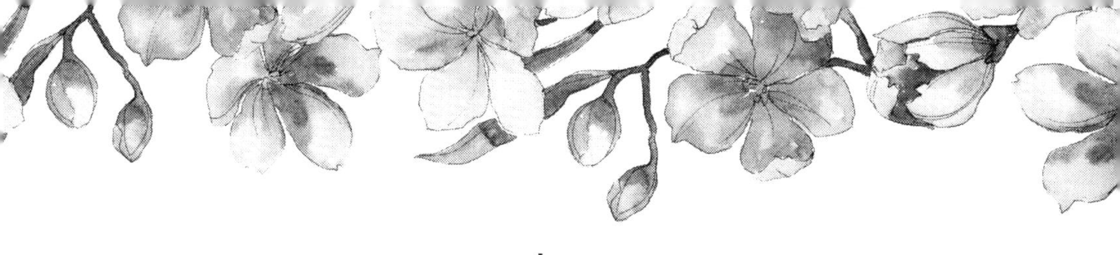

WEEK 12 | RECAP

HOW HAS THIS WEEK BEEN FOR YOU?

IN WHAT WAYS HAVE YOU GROWN?

HOW DO YOU FEEL NOW AFTER WORKING YOUR WAY THROUGH THIS JOURNAL?

NOTES

NOTES

NOTES

NOTES

Made in the USA
Columbia, SC
22 February 2024